This book is to be returned on or before the last date stamped below.

2 1 AUG 1985

HUESTON & TUBIANA

No. 1. Copy

DUPUYTREN'S DISEASE

Monographs of the Group d'Etude de la Main
Series edited by R. Tubiana

GROUPE D'ETUDE DE LA MAIN (G.E.M.)
List of members

DUPUYTREN'S DISEASE

Edited by J. T. Hueston and R. Tubiana

in collaboration with
E. Benassayag J. M. Bruner R. M. Curtis
G. Fisk R. I. Gonzalez J. Gosset W. Hakstian
F. Iselin M. Iselin J. I. P. James
J. W. Littler C. R. McCash J. Michon
H. Millesi C. Nézelof M. Shaw
T. Skoog H. G. Stack J.-M. Thomine

First English edition

CHURCHILL LIVINGSTONE Edinburgh and London 1974

CHURCHILL LIVINGSTONE

Medical Division of Longman Group Limited

Represented in the United States of America by
Longman Inc., New York and by associated
companies, branches and representatives throughout
the world.

First edition, Second edition (in French)
© Expansion Scientifique Française 1966, 1972

Third edition (in English)
© Longman Group Ltd. 1974

ISBN 0 443 01048 X

Preface to the English Edition

Originally based on 1966 S.I.C.O.T. Papers presented in Paris and expanded by invited French and Foreign contributors to this subject, this volume was first produced by the Groupe d'Etude de la Main as a record of the current opinions on the controversial subject of Dupuytren's disease. Embodying as they did a diversity of opinion and creating an authentic atmosphere of sincere scientific discussion the first two editions were mainly in French with English summaries and have proved so successful as to stimulate this present English language Third Edition.

This present volume has been entirely produced in English to lessen the bulk of a bilingual book and has included further contributions, both English and French. The colourful Patrick Clarkson was so popular at the Paris Meeting of the Groupe d'Etude de la Main in 1964 that a posthumous gesture of including his work was suggested by my colleague Raoul Tubiana.

Neither editor has dictated policy to the contributors. Much of Gallic flavour has survived into the English renditions. Thus while retaining its G.E.M. quality it is hoped that this potpourri of papers will keep alive the interest and enthusiasm of surgeons seeking to solve the enigma of Dupuytren's disease.

Compared to the 1966 papers a definite alignment of opinion is beginning to emerge and perhaps a later edition may be able to present the total solution to this problem disease.

In the meantime it is important to keep alive our interest and intellectual activity. It is hoped that this collection of papers helps to do so!

Acknowledgements

The editors are grateful to Mr W. F. Wilson, F.R.A.C.S., for his assistance in compiling the index to the English edition.

Article No. 10, entitled 'Observations on Dupuytren's Disease' by the late Patrick Clarkson, has been reprinted from *Clinical Surgery*, vol. 7, 'The Hand', pp. 229–233, ed. Charles Rob and Rodney Smith; London: Butterworth, 1966, and is reproduced by kind permission of the publishers.

JOHN HUESTON

Preface to the Second Edition

This new edition is very different from that which appeared in 1966.

The papers originally presented at a Round Table of the Congress of the Societe Internationale de Chirurgie Orthopedique et de Traumatologie (S.I.C.O.T.) have been brought together again in this second edition. However, as Professor Jean Gosset—who was chairman of the Round Table—said in his introduction to the first edition: the papers presented 'could not pretend to represent a complete monograph or even a balanced view of the treatment of Dupuytren's contracture. The authors have only tackled the current problems and expressed their own opinions and their management'. Not only have these earlier texts been completely revised and often considerably enlarged by the authors but we are endeavouring to show a much wider and more varied picture of this strange and fascinating 'maladie'. A glance through the Table of Contents would show that the number of articles has been doubled and include anatomy, histology, aetiology, clinical aspects and various forms of treatment of this condition.

I am afraid, however, that despite this abundance of papers the reader will not be entirely satisfied or may even be slightly confused by this very same abundance. It is stressed that there is no aspect of what Dr M. Iselin has appropriately termed 'this mysterious disease' which does not deserve continuing discussion and investigation.

Moreover, in this abundance of hypotheses and often contradictory opinions some points of agreement can be found, which offer hope that we are approaching the point where therapeutic logic and scientific truth can finally come to terms.

Those responsible for this present monograph, John Hueston and myself, have tried to effect such a synthesis between the aetiological studies and therapeutic procedures. Work currently in progress will inevitably require another stocktaking and evaluation sooner or later. It is precisely this role which we hope is filled by this series of monographs from the Groupe d'Etude de la Main.

This edition introduces a new policy of publication by G.E.M. Rather than group together both the French and English versions of each article in a single volume we will in future be publishing a separate monograph in each of the two languages. This of course often will require two editors with one responsible for each of the language editions. We hope that the co-editors of those several monographs in preparation have as profitable and friendly a collaboration as John Hueston and I have enjoyed.

RAOUL TUBIANA
Secretary General of G.E.M.

List of Contributors

E. BENASSAYAG Clinique Urologique, Hôpital Cochin, 27, fg Saint-Jaques, 75-Paris 14, France

J. M. BRUNER 1005 Banker's Trust Building, Des Moines, Iowa 50309, U.S.A.

R. M. CURTIS 2947 St Paul Street, Baltimore, Maryland 21218, U.S.A.

G. FISK The Mount, Debden Green, Loughton, Essex, United Kingdom

R. I. GONZALEZ 101 San Mateo Drive, San Mateo, California 94410, U.S.A.

J. GOSSET 86 rue d'Assas, 75-Paris 06, France

R. W. HAKSTIAN Drummond Medical Building, Drummond Street, Montreal, Canada

J. T. HUESTON 89 Royal Parade, Parkville, Melbourne, Australia

F. ISELIN 1 rue Auguste-Vacquerie, 75-Paris 16, France

M. ISELIN 1 rue Auguste-Vacquerie, 75-Paris 16, France

J. I. P. JAMES Department of Orthopaedic Surgery, University of Edinburgh, United Kingdom

J. W. LITTLER 14 East 90th Street, New York 28, U.S.A.

C. R. McCASH Honorary Consultant Plastic Surgeon, Westminster Hospital, London, United Kingdom

J. MICHON Hôpital Jeanne-d'Arc, 54 Dommartin-les-Touls, France

H. MILLESI Chirurgische Universitätsklinik, Alser Strasse 4, 1090 Vienna, Austria

C. NEZELOF 27 rue Gazan, 75-Paris 14, France

M. SHAW 20 Clarendon Road, Leeds 2, United Kingdom

T. SKOOG Akademiska Sjukhuset, Uppsala, Sweden

H. G. STACK Westhay, Mount Avenue, Hutton, Essex, United Kingdom

J.-M. THOMINE 7 rue du Vert-Buisson, 76-Rouen, France

R. TUBIANA 47 quai des Grands-Augustins, 75-Paris 06, France

Foreword

BARON DUPUYTREN, P.-L. Chigot

With his slender refined nose, small and even scornful mouth, stock neck in Restoration lace arising out of a fashionable frock coat and vest, we have the man of the fracture, the contraction of the palmar aponeurosis, the enterotome, and the Museum—Baron Dupuytren.

In 1818, aged 40 years, his years' surgical output was impressive; he performed 378 operations, reduced 178 fractures and opened 300 abscesses; 2363 patients were admitted to hospital and of the 378 patients operated 228 were cured, in other words 5 patients out of 8. Certainly an extraordinary performance in an era which can hardly be described as aseptic.

It is often claimed that he was the first to discover the retraction of the palmar aponeurosis and that this was in his own coachman. In fact the condition had already been recognized by Astley Cooper in England and Boyer in France both of whom had declared the condition to be incurable.

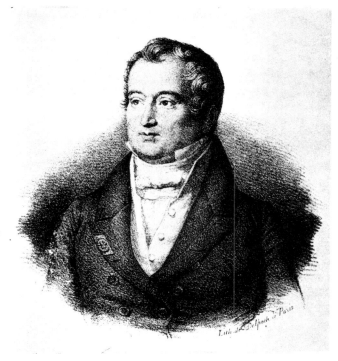

But three facts gave Dupuytren the opportunity to immortalize his name eponymously.

On the 5th December 1831 he announced to his class that he would speak 'of only one patient and of only one disease'. The patient was a 40 year old coachman, Demarteau, from bed 63 in Saint Marthe's Ward in the Hôtel Dieu.

Dupuytren presented the symptoms in a description that we still use after 100 years. Then in the same lesson he presented his own dissection of the hand of an old man with this condition and demonstrated that neither the tendons nor the skin were the cause of the deformity but that essentially this was due to the retraction of the palmar aponeurosis.

Finally after these clinical and anatomical dissertations he demonstrated his first attempt at operative correction. Since 1811 he had reviewed a patient Emil in whom the contracture had continued to progress so that on 12 June 1831 he had operated. Without anaesthetic he had made a transverse incision one inch long opposite the metacarpophalangeal joint of the ring finger, then a second incision opposite the little finger and a third across the middle of the proximal phalanx. The palmar aponeurosis was incised 'with a clearly audible crack'. The fingers came out straight and dressings were applied. Healing was completed on the 2nd of July and an extension splint was applied until the 2nd of August.

'Today 5th December 1831, the patient is perfectly healed' and to conclude the session Dupuytren proceeded to operate on Demarteau, who was neither his coachman nor his first patient and not even his first operated case.

Our Baron wrote very little apart from a huge collection of observations made at the Hôtel Dieu and recorded in 100 large folio volumes.

The lecture notes religiously recorded by his students, Briere de Boismont, Paillard and Marx, filled five volumes. The entire 500 pages of the first volume of these lecture notes are entirely devoted to a study of traumatic and inflammatory lesions of the locomotor system.

His ability, force and capacity for astute yet prudent clinical decisions, were to be found side by side with a most ruthless ambition and unscrupulous nature.

His treatment of his teacher Pellatan whose position he sought at the Hôtel Dieu has been severely criticized. He has also been accused of having plagiarized much of the pathology treatise of Bichart soon after the author's death. Laennec was so disturbed by Dupuytren's dishonesty that he disassociated himself and opened a separate teaching school of pathology.

In his defence his students, however, claimed 'such defects can be excused if on behalf of humanity the work is pursued with such almost religious dedication'.

At 68 years he developed pleurisy during a meeting of the Faculty of Medicine and died in a few days while Cruveilher, Bouillaud and Broussais were debating whether to drain his empyema. In Dupuytren's opinion if was 'better to die of the disease than of the operation'!

Replete with honours and titles, so rich that he could offer a million francs to help the exiled King Charles X, his reputation was enormous. In that romantic era, the day of his funeral in 1835 was long recalled—colleagues and scholars having come from all over the country. His mortal remains were carried to Pere-LaChaise by his students who would not delegate this last duty to anyone else.

Finally, glancing through the *Lancette Français* of 1831, we find his writings on 'Nepotism', 'Reform of the medical course', 'On the ignorance of teachers'—after all the burial of a Mandarin is always a grand and satisfying ceremony!

Contents

Preface to the English edition v

Preface to the second edition *R. Tubiana* vii

List of Contributors viii

Foreword: Baron Dupuytren *P.-L. Chigot* ix

1. The development and anatomy of the digital fascia *J.-M. Thomine* 1
2. Dupuytren's disease and the anatomy of the palmodigital aponeuroses *J. Gosset* 11
3. Histological aspects of Dupuytren's contracture *C. Nézelof* 25
4. Aetiological questions in Dupuytren's contracture *J. T. Hueston* 29
5. The genetic pattern of Dupuytren's contracture and idiopathic epilepsy *J. I. P. James* 37
6. The relationship of trauma to Dupuytren's contracture *G. Fisk* 43
7. Evaluation of deformity in Dupuytren's contracture *R. Tubiana, J. Michon and J.-M. Thomine* 45
8. The clinical and morphological course of Dupuytren's disease *H. Millesi* 49
9. Prognosis as a guide to the timing and extent of surgery in Dupuytren's contracture *J. T. Hueston* 61
10. Observations on Dupuytren's disease *P. Clarkson* 63
11. Mysterious aspects of Dupuytren's contracture *M. Iselin* 67
12. The principles of surgical treatment of Dupuytren's contracture *R. Tubiana* 71
13. Late results of extensive fasciectomy *R. W. Hakstian* 79
14. Surgical treatment of Dupuytren's contracture: technique of fasciotomy and fasciectomy *R. Tubiana and J.-M. Thomine* 85
15. Technique of selective aponeurectomy for Dupuytren's contracture *J. M. Bruner* 93
16. Some practical points in the surgical treatment of Dupuytren's contracture *M. Shaw* 95
17. Special points of technique in Dupuytren's contracture *J. W. Littler* 97
18. Operative difficulties and postoperative complications in the surgery of Dupuytren's contracture *J. Michon* 101
19. Dupuytren's contracture: pathogenesis and surgical treatment *T. Skoog* 109
20. Skin replacement in Dupuytren's contracture *J. T. Hueston* 119
21. Open fasciotomy and full thickness skin graft in the correction of digital flexion deformity *R. I. Gonzalez* 123
22. The open palm technique in Dupuytren's contracture *C. R. McCash* 129
23. Volar capsulectomy of the proximal interphalangeal joint in Dupuytren's contracture *R. M. Curtis* 135
24. Recurrences in Dupuytren's contracture *F. Iselin* 139
25. Enzymic fasciotomy *J. T. Hueston* 141
26. The management of ectopic lesions in Dupuytren's contracture *J. T. Hueston* 145
27. The treatment of Peyronie's disease by methylhydrazine *E. Benassayag* 149
28. The palmar fascia, and the development of deformities and displacements in Dupuytren's contracture *H. G. Stack* 153
29. Points of agreement and modern trends in the treatment of Dupuytren's contracture *R. Tubiana* 163

Author index 165

Subject index 165

1. THE DEVELOPMENT AND ANATOMY OF THE DIGITAL FASCIA

Jean-Michel Thomine

This present study is based on two series of investigations. The first has been carried out under the supervision of Professor J. M. F. Landsmeer in the Anatomy Department of the University of Leyden and involved the study of serial sections 10 μ thick from foetal hands ranging in age from 15 to 18 weeks (foetal length 11·5 to 14 cm) except for one of 25 weeks intrauterine life. Actually the study of serial sections of the hand, so difficult in adults, is relatively straightforward in the human foetus. It allows the recognition, by 15 weeks of intrauterine life, of an aponeurotic layer which it is reasonable to regard as the pattern of later development of the fascial structures of the hand.

The second part of this work is the macroscopic anatomy and is based on the dissection of 20 hands; two from a 1-year old subject and the other 18 from the dissecting rooms of the Faculty of Medicine in Paris (Professor A. Delmas). The age and sex of these patients could not be recorded. The side does not seem to have been an important factor.

The technique of dissection has been important. The skinning of the hand has been first performed as superficially as possible, before beginning the deeper dissection. This is simple enough on the dorsum where the skin is mobile and easily detached. It is much more difficult on the palmar aspect where, throughout its width, the deep aspect of the dermis is bound to the superficial aspect of the aponeurotic sheet by a multitude of tiny fibrous strands which enclose the loculi of subdermal fat. This produces a remarkable fixation of the palmar skin and explains the anatomical interdependence between the skin and the fibrous structures

of the hand. On dividing the dermal attachment of these fibrous strands it is possible to remove only the skin leaving the contours of the skinned hand undisturbed. It is also easy to recognize certain zones of direct adherence of the skin to the deeper structures and these will be pointed out later.

The following points will be considered:

The distribution of the fibrous envelopes of the fingers which for convenience will be called the 'digital fascia'.

The relation of the digital fascia to the overlying skin and with the deeper structures.

Its relation with the palmar fibrous structures, where particular attention will be paid to the natatory ligament of the web space.

Variations found in certain areas, the lateral border of the index, medial border of the little finger the thumb and the first web space.

THE FIBROUS ENVELOPES OF THE FINGERS

Neither in the adult nor in the foetus can the digital fascia be regarded as similar in thickness or structure to the fascia of the forearm or the palm. The only structure which can be followed continuously from the web space to the base of the distal phalanx is the fibrous sheath of the neurovascular bundles. Distribution in the foetal hand (Figs. 1.1, 1.2, 1.3) shows how this condensation will be laid down in the adult (Fig. 1.6).

The volar part of the digital fascia which interests us most here is literally laid down around the neuro-

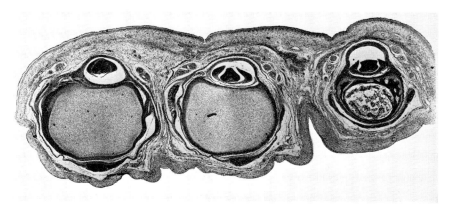

Figure 1.1
Foetal hand: transverse section through 3rd and 4th web space, showing from left to right the splitting of the investing digital fascia to enclose the neurovascular bundles.

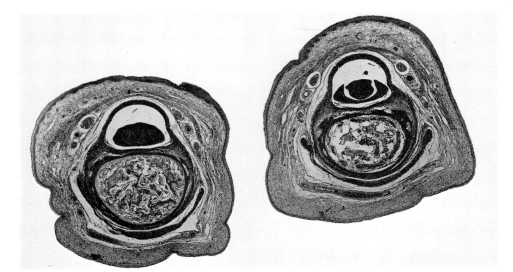

Figure 1.2
Foetal hand: transverse section through the middle of 2 proximal phalanges showing the condensation of fibres from the natatory ligaments reinforcing the lateral and the posterior border of each neurovascular sheath.

vascular bundles. From the palm to the distal interphalangeal joint the neurovascular bundles run on the anterolateral aspect of the fibrous flexor tendon sheath, each bundle being enclosed in the condensation first seen at the web space level, and showing in section an elliptical outline with its long axis oblique to both the volar plane and the axis of the finger. Each sheath consists of a superficial layer and a deep layer which fuse together again in front and behind the bundle on the midline of the finger; between the volar pole of these

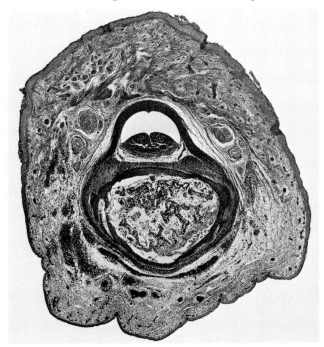

Figure 1.3
Foetal hand: transverse section of a middle phalanx showing the posterolateral bundle of fibres reinforcing the neurovascular sheath.

two ellipses the digital fascia has only one layer which unites the two sheaths.

The volar digital fascia takes on the appearance of a cloak thrown over the flexor tendon sheath.

The posterior pole of each ellipse lies almost level with the lateral margin of the phalanx. It is continuous behind with the dorsal fascia which forms a single layer covering the superficial aspect of the extensor apparatus. The structure of the digital fascia can thus be regarded schematically as forming a simple circular sheath enclosing bone and tendons and splitting on the anterolateral aspect of the finger to enclose the neurovascular bundles. But the neurovascular sheath itself has a peculiar relationship with the deeper structures of the finger and with the palmar fascia and thus retains the greatest significance in the digital fascia.

The deep layer of the neurovascular sheath is transparent and tenuous. The superficial layer appears thicker but is more difficult to dissect because of its connection with the fibrous strands joining it to the skin through the fatty layer.

It must be emphasized that there exists at the level of the posterior angle of the elliptical neurovascular sheath, that is in the plane of the lateral border of the phalanges, a more resistant zone of a denser fibrous tissue than anywhere else in the digital fascia. This is recognizable in the foetal hand sections (Figs. 1.1, 1.2, 1.3). Less well defined in the proximal segment of the finger, this posterior condensation is seen there as a fine network after removing the neurovascular bundle; in the middle segment it becomes a strong fibrous bundle exceeding one millimetre in diameter. It will thus be known by the name of 'retrovascular band' (Fig. 7). Its relations with the deep structures of the fingers in the aponeurotic elements of the palm are of great interest.

Thus defined the digital fascia stops at the level of

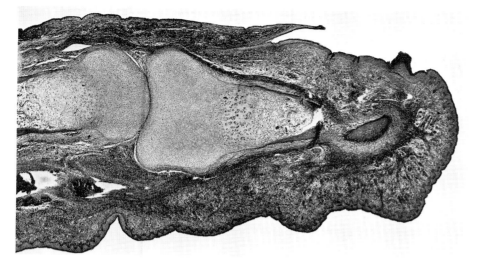

the distal interphalangeal joint. Dorsally it gives place to the nailbed and on the volar aspect its layers disappear as such to allow the formation of the nervous and vascular endings in the pulp. The only recognizable fibrous structures in the distal segment of the finger are the strands dividing up the subdermal fat into loculi and here binding the skin directly to the underlying periosteum of the distal phalanx. A sagittal section of the foetal pulp demonstrates this arrangement (Fig. 1.4).

RELATIONS OF THE DIGITAL FASCIA TO THE OVERLYING SKIN

The loose union between dorsal skin and dorsal fascia except for the distal phalanx, and the fibrous mesh which fixes the volar and subcutaneous fatty layer have already been described. Two other zones need special description.

(*a*) At the flexure creases the subcutaneous fatty layers becomes very attenuated and disappears and the skin is directly fixed to the digital fascia.

(*b*) An analogous zone of direct adherence exists at the line of junction of dorsal and palmar skin all along the finger. At the base of the proximal segment it is strictly linear and merges into the plane of the web space crest. Beyond this level the zone of direct contact between skin and fascia appears as a large strip of strong adhesion. All this zone of adhesion projects a little beyond the neurovascular bundle and thus corresponds to the retrovascular band.

RELATIONS OF THE DIGITAL FASCIA TO THE DEEP STRUCTURES OF THE FINGER

Concerning these relations the following points must be noted:

Freedom of movement of the dorsal fascia on the underlying structure.

At the volar aspect the contrast between the free median zone and the lateral zones where the deeper aspect of the digital fascia acquires its fixation.

Indeed, if the median volar sheet of the digital fascia which unites the neurovascular bundles is incised longitudinally, a plane of cleavage is exposed between its deep surface and the superficial surface of the fibrous

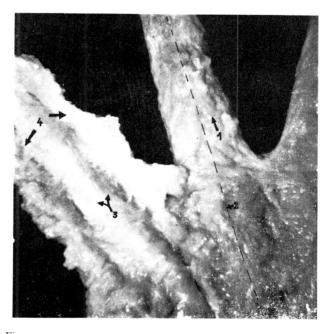

Figure 1.5
The digital fascia: (1) skin only removed; (2) line of incision for exposure of; (3) the pretendinous plane of cleavage, and (4) the 2 halves of the palmar digital fascia reflected laterally.

from Cleland's is offered. This band is not considered as a roughly transverse osteocutaneous ligament but as a longitudinal structure with points of elective fixation to the skeleton—the base of the proximal phalanges and interphalangeal joint levels—and having an important continuity with certain volar structures of which the most important is the natatory ligament. The superficial skin fixation and the deep skeletal fixation of the retrovascular band can be destroyed without its losing its identity.

Moreover the total absence of any transverse structure in the foetus contrasts with the fibrous condensations

ANTERIORLY

The digital vessels and nerves lose first their dense fascial protection at the distal border of the superficial transverse palmar ligament. In the intervening region they are covered by a fine connective tissue. Such a slight covering layer also exists in front of the proximal part of the pulleys of the tendon sheath—after the termination of the pretendinous bundle mainly by insertion on the deeper aspect of the skin.

All the present studies have confirmed this abrupt termination of the palmar fascial structures at this level

flexor tendon sheath. On section this semicircular space is seen to contain only a very loose areolar network; it is better defined over the proximal segment than over the middle segment; of course it disappears over the distal segment (Fig. 1.5).

This volar space is quite separated from the dorsal space by a series of lateral structures located along the side of the phalanges (Fig. 1.6).

At first there are strong adhesions of the deeper aspect of the neurovascular sheath and then of the retrovascular band to the proximal segment of the retinacular ligament extending for several millimetres in the palmar–dorsal direction. After dividing these adhesions there appears a very peculiar organization of the retrovascular fibrous band and of its relations with the retinacular ligament. The retrovascular band to the proximal phalanx joins that of the second phalanx after the zone of adhesion to the retinacular ligament. But it appears that at the second phalanx the retrovascular band is seen as a strong fibrous bundle with a bony attachment at the

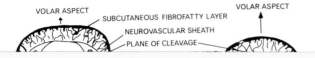

(Fig. 1.11); this fascial hiatus separating the true palmar aponeurosis and the natatory ligament is easily seen on sections of the foetal hand (Fig. 1.1).

THE NATATORY LIGAMENT (FIG. 1.10)

Its superior and proximal border extends onto the proximal phalanges and follows an almost straight line from the lateral border of the index to the medial border of the little finger. In front of each tendon sheath it fuses with a thin fascial layer already described; in the web space it is outlined by the fatty lobules of the region.

Its inferior or distal border naturally is different as it corresponds to the beginning of the finger or to the web space.

At the base of the finger it fuses with the digital fascia so that in the midline of the finger it is in continuity with the median sheet which it reinforces over the front of the proximal phalanx. Laterally it is continuous with the superficial sheet of the neurovascular bundle.

In each web space the natatory ligament has a slightly oblique plane, its proximal border being more volar than its distal—so that it forms an anterior slope of what can be called the 'commissural roof'; the posterior surface is a thin dorsal fascia (Fig. 1.10). This fascia and the natatory ligament fuse at the end of the web

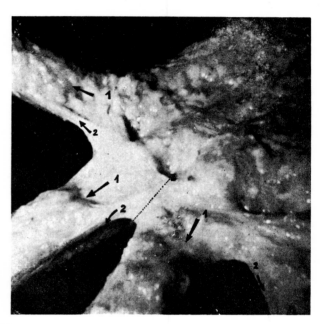

Figure 1.11
A, Distal palmar dissection showing (1) continuity of palmar ligament with digital fascia and (2) the fibres of origin of the web space which reinforce it.

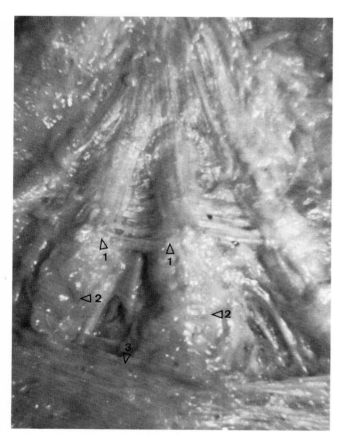

Figure 1.10
Distal palm showing the aponeurotic hiatus: (1) A difference in texture occurs at the distal end of the pretendinous band; (2) The thin covering over the flexor tendons and their hollow; (3) The proximal border of the interdigital palmar ligament.

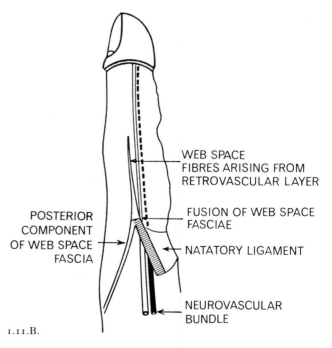

1.11.B.

to form the 'commissural crest'. The 'commissural roof' has two gables which extend onto the side of the adjacent fingers and one may notice that because of its obliquity the proximal border of the natatory ligament is in the superficial plane of the palm so that its distal border corresponds to the line of junction of the dorsal and palmar skin of the finger. The 'commissural crest' is prolonged by a visible bundle of fibres along most of the proximal phalangeal segment. Some of these fibres reinforce the posterior part of a superficial layer of the neurovascular sheath; the deepest are in the retrovascular position and contribute to the retrovascular fibrous band.

LATERALLY

After the bifurcation in the distal palm the digital neurovascular bundles lie close beside the sagittal paratendinous septum which shows the same attenuation as the other volar fascial structures at the distal part of the palm. Indeed after the important deep extensions of the palmar aponeurosis have ceased, it is only represented by a weak fibrous sheath. Only a few significant longitudinal fibres are found in this layer which seems separate from the pretendinous band of the palmar aponeurosis. These fibres pass very deeply almost to the level of the deep fascia and contribute further to the retrovascular fibrous band. This sagittal paratendinous layer, already medial to the neurovascular bundle is continued in the finger with the deep layer of the retrovascular sheath.

POSTERIORLY

The neurovascular bundle at first rests on the deep fascia of the palm either directly or by the intermediate action of the lumbrical muscle covered by the fibrous layer of the canals of Legueu and Juvara. It is from these retrovascular structures that the last elements of the retrovascular fibrous band of the finger are derived. Numerous weak fibres extend frontally from the deep fascial plane of the palm as well as from the fascial sheath of the lumbrical.

The fibres nearest the digital axis form the posterior aspect of the neurovascular sheath contributing to the neurovascular band. Others join the deep aspect of the apex of the 'commissural roof' fixing it and separating the dorsal from the volar subfascial spaces.

Thus the digital neurovascular sheath is formed on its lateral aspect from elements of the paratendinous septum and on its superficial aspect from elements of the natatory ligament. These two parts remain separate in the web space and the posterior aspect of the sheath only becomes closed at the finger level. The retrovascular band is formed from three sets of fibres in the proximal phalangeal segment. Most fibres come from the web space fibres passing behind the vessels. Fewest fibres come from the pretendinous band through the

paratendinous sheath and the third contribution comes from a continuation of the deep fascial plane of the palm (Fig. 1.12).

The fascial continuity from the palm into the finger is thus made in its strongest part by these retrovascular elements continuing as the retrovascular fibrous band.

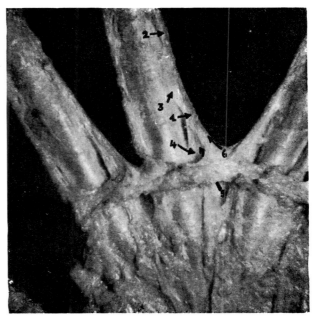

Figure 1.12
Distal palm with removal of all digital fascia except the retrovascular band whose main attachments have been preserved, namely (1) the fine band to the proximal phalanx; (2) the fibrous bundle which it forms on the middle phalangeal segment; (3) the bony attachment at the level of the proximal interphalangeal joint; (4) attachment to the base of proximal segment; (5) contribution from the deep aponeurosis; (6) the web space fibres of the natatory ligament.

This continuity exists in the superficial volar plane by means of the weak sheath covering the tendons, vessels and nerves between the palmar aponeurosis itself and the natatory ligament. In the sagittal plane there is only the feeble remains of the paratendinous septum.

This general account requires modification in four special areas:

1. *The thumb.* The digital fascia of the thumb is rendered unique because of the relative independence between the digital and palmar fascia, the existence of only two phalanges, the absence of the fibrous flexor sheath in the palm, and the single origin of the two neurovascular pedicles. Roughly a detachment is at the proximal phalangeal level that of the ordinary finger and at the distal phalangeal that of the ordinary distal phalanx. However, these fibrous structures are denser along the radial aspect of the thumb and are usually

fixed to the collateral ligament of the interphalangeal joint. On the other hand the thumb fascia is not reinforced from the palm or the web space and the retrovascular bundle is poorly defined. Finally the continuity between the superficial layer, the neurovascular bundles and the weak thenar fascia is virtually the only connection between the palmar and digital fascia of this digit.

2. *The index.* On the lateral margin of this finger can be noted (a) the very large and dense adhesion of the skin to the digital fascia on the dorso-palmar junctional line which extends only slightly into the first web space; (b) a particularly dense lateral retrovascular band; (c) the extremely weak contribution of longitudinal fibres from the corresponding paratendinous septum.

3. *The little finger.* This also shows strong cutaneous fixation along the medial dorso-palmar digital line and this is continued onto the ulnar border of the hand. The medial retrovascular band is denser and more firmly bound to the deeper structures. No fibres from the paratendinous septa appear to contribute to it. Specific connections are seen between the medial neurovascular digital sheath and the abductor digiti minimi muscle. The retrovascular bundle is so fused with its tendon that sharp dissection is required to separate them while the superficial layer of the bundle is in continuity with the fascia covering the belly of the muscle. Finally the natatory ligament at this level splits as it reaches the medial border of the little finger; the posterior layer passing behind the neurovascular bundle and reaching the bone anterior to the insertion of the abductor digiti minimi, while the superficial layer passes over the neurovascular bundle to fuse with the tendon of the same muscle and finally to be inserted behind its tendon on the medial border of the proximal phalanx.

Some analogy exists between the medial aspect of the little finger and the lateral aspect of the index where the lumbrical corresponds to the abductor—the natatory ligament does not fuse with the lumbrical tendon and a sheet joining the two fascial layers separates the tendon from the vessels.

4. *The first web space.* The special fascial arrangements here are due to the large and mobile muscle mass of the web space and the thenar eminence and the absence of the deep transverse ligaments of the palm. The fascial covering is only represented by the sheaths of the muscles which in turn are continuous with the digital fascia of the thumb laterally and the index medially.

The most lateral longitudinal fibres of the palmar aponeurosis and the most lateral transverse fibres of the superficial transverse ligament of the palm extend into the deep aspect of the skin of the web space, but lie superficial to the fascial envelope of the muscles. Apart from these fibres there is little connection between skin and fascia in this region. Finally one must emphasise the absence of arciform fibres in the first web space, in the apex of which there is a direct fusion between dorsal and palmar skin.

CONCLUSION AND SURGICAL SIGNIFICANCE

Dupuytren's contracture and its treatment is first and foremost concerned with the local anatomy.

The binding between web space and digital structures explains the lack of fingers spreading frequently associated with their lack of extension. The aponeurotic cord frequently seen at the medial side of the base of the fifth finger has been found to have an anatomical origin. The variable position of the neurovascular pedicles regarding the digital cords can be explained by variable location of the disease in the digital fascia and specially in the neurovascular sheath.

It is noteworthy that those zones among the most severely affected by fascial contractures—the distal part of the paratendinous septa, near the base of the finger—are among those areas least well supplied by dense fascial components and almost corresponding to a fascial hiatus.

It is the same in the finger where the contracture is not always along the line of the retrovascular band but in the thinner anterior region.

The same again is seen in the first web space where a strong fascial network is not normally found.

Perhaps the exact site of origin of the fibrous lesions should be re-examined in the light of these observations.

Finally the specific relationship between the skin and the deeper structures over the whole extent of the volar aspect of the hand should be borne in mind.

To end on a specific technical point, it is noted that a plane of cleavage exists deep to the volar sheet of the digital fascia and by dissection in this plane the vitality of the skin flaps is preserved while the exposure of the neurovascular bundles is facilitated.

REFERENCES

CLELAND, J. (1878). On the cutaneous ligaments of the phalange. *Journal of Anatomy and Physiology*, p. 526 and plate XVII.

JAMES, J. & TUBIANA, R. (1952). La maladie de Dupuytren. *Revue de Chirurgie orthopédique et réparatrice de l'Appareil moteur*, **38,** 352.

KANAVEL, A. B., KOCH, S. L. & MASON, M. L. (1929). Dupuytren's contracture. *Surgery, Gynecology and Obstetrics*, **48,** 145.

KAPLAN, E. B. (1938). The palmar fascia in connection with Dupuytren's contracture. *Surgery*, **4,** 415–422.

KEMPF, I. & GONZALO-VIVAR, F. (1963). Les formations fibro-aponévrotiques de la région métacarpo-phalangienne. *Comptes rendus de l'Association des anatomistes,* 48th reunion, no. 118, 804–814.

LANDSMEER, J. M. F. (1948). The anatomy of the dorsal aponeurosis of the human finger and its functional significance. *Anatomical Record,* **104,** 35–45.

LEGUEU, F. & JUVARA, E. (1892). Des aponévroses de la paume de la main. *Bulletin de la Societe anatomique*, Paris, 67, 5th series, T. VI.

LEROUX (1958). Contribution a l'etude de la maladie de Dupuytren. Thesis, Paris.

MASLIEURAT-LAGEMARD (1839). Sur l'anatomie descriptive et chirurgicale des aponévroses et membranes synoviales de la main, de leur application a la thérapeutique et a la médecine operatoire. *Gazette medicale, Paris,* 273.

MILFORD, L. W. (1968). *Retaining Ligaments of the Digits of the Hand.* Philadelphia: Saunders.

STACK, G. (1961). Anatomy of the fascia of the fingers. *The Second Hand Club Meeting in Gothenburg.* Copenhagen: Malmo.

THOMINE, J. M. (1965). Conjonctif d'enveloppe des doigts et squelette fibreux des commissures interdigitales. *Annales de Chirurgie plastique,* **3,** 194–203.

TUBIANA, R. (1964). Le traitement sélectif de la maladie de Dupuytren. *Revue de Chirurgie orthopédique et réparatrice de l'Appareil moteur,* **50,** 311–334.

2. DUPUYTREN'S DISEASE AND THE ANATOMY OF THE PALMODIGITAL APONEUROSES

J. Gosset

Baron Boyer stepped into immortality by claiming, around 1830, that surgery had reached the limit of its possibilities. Another of his unfortunate phrases was 'crispatura tendinum', which he used in describing the hand lesion which results in fixed flexion of the fingers. Dupuytren dissecting one such hand found bands which ran *alongside* the affected fingers. In 1832, he found that a retraction of the aponeurosis was in fact the main lesion in the disease which later was to bear his name. According to J. Windsor, Henry Cline demonstrated (as early as 1808) the favourable effect of fasciotomy and Astley Cooper in 1822 followed Cline's example. Does this mean that Dupuytren's fame is undeserved? Whatever the case may be, he believed that the disease was the result of trauma and that it attacked the aponeurotic structures.

But in 1834, Goyrand challenged these two facts. He denied that trauma was the main ætiological factor, and claimed that the retractile fibrous structures which cause fixed flexion of the fingers are independent of both the palmar aponeurosis and the tendons.

On the first point, Goyrand might well have been right. The real ætiology of Dupuytren's disease remains a mystery.

Must we now challenge Dupuytren's theory on the second point as well? This is just what Hueston has done in an important work published in 1963. According to this Australian surgeon, the nodules and the fibrous bands excised are quite separate from the palmar aponeurosis. In fact he believes them to be new fibrous formations, developing initially between the skin and the aponeurosis. They arise from none of the recognized anatomical structures, and constitute what he calls 'Dupuytren's tissue'.

As a result, surgical excision should not be determined by anatomical factors—a fact which rather indicates limited or selective resections.

Is this opinion wholly or partially true? This we would like to discuss as it is of primary importance to the surgeon.

If the lesions are independent new-formations, unrelated to the recognized anatomical elements, their excision will be haphazard and will be concentrated on avoiding neurovascular structures. If on the contrary the lesions develop in a well defined anatomical structure, e.g. the digitopalmar aponeurosis, their excision will be carried out in a systematic, orderly way. There will

be no unexpected anomalies, and only the uninitiated will have unpleasant surprises.

We must see first how much can be learned from microscopical examination. In this respect the works of Meyerding, and those of Nezeloff and Tubiana are precise and tend to agree. These authors have shown that two very different types of lesions are encountered in Dupuytren's disease.

In some areas, one finds fibroblastic activity, mitoses, little collagen, a disorderly arrangement with wavy or concentric patterns. In others, there is a paucity of cells, dense collagen arranged in parallel fibres and forming actual retractile bands.

One may accept the theory, proposed by a number of authors, that the first type of lesion represents the early, progressive stage of the disease, while the other represents a late, stabilized stage. As this theory has never yet been confirmed, we feel free to suggest an alternative one: the cellular, nodular lesion and the collagen bands are two forms of the same disease occurring in different structures.

The acellular, collagenous forms are very retractile, and are the ones responsible for flexion of the metacarpophalangeal and interphalangeal joints. They lead to the formation of fibrous bands over which the skin of the palm remains thin, supple and mobile, except for a few millimetres proximal and distal to the flexion creases.

The nodular forms of Dupuytren's disease are quite different. Histologically, they present as a dense tissue, rich in cells and showing no organization. The picture is the same in the palmar and digital nodules, in the knuckle pads and in the plantar nodules of Ledderhose. In the hand, the round or oval shaped nodules adhere closely to the skin which becomes callous over the lesions. These are pretendinous and are usually found in areas where the fatty tissue is thick, between the interphalangeal creases, between the proximal I.P. and the M.P. creases, and only rarely proximal to this.

In our experience, as we shall see later, the nodules usually form in areas where no aponeurotic structure would be found in the normal hand. They are but slightly retractile. If after the removal of a large phalangeal nodule the finger still does not achieve complete extension, it is essential to look elsewhere (and we shall see where) for a band the severing of which will ensure a good result. Depending on the cases, any combination of these two distinct forms may be encountered. Some cases are primarily nodular, and flexion is not pronounced. In other cases, the nodules are virtually absent and the strongly retractile bands prevail. Type D of the disease, described by Michon and Tubiana, is characterized by the presence of these bands which we shall describe later. And finally, there are cases where both forms are encountered, in equal or unequal proportions.

We believe that the bands and nodules do not represent two different stages in the course of the disease, but rather two distinct forms, which originate in different tissues. When the disease develops in a well defined sheet of aponeurosis, the lesion takes the form of dense, retracted fibrous bands, with abundant collagen and a paucity of cells. When it affects the adipose tissue, and spares the aponeurosis, the nodular form prevails. The fat disappears, the cellular fibrosis invades the deep layer of the skin and spreads inwards towards the underlying aponeurosis. In other words, we believe that the two forms which differ macroscopically (nodules or bands) and histologically, represent lesions in different tissues: in the fatty tissue for the nodules, and in the aponeurosis for the bands.

We agree with Hueston's view that the nodular lesion is independent of the aponeurosis. It shows a preference for the pretendinous zones where there is no aponeurosis, at the base of the phalanx, distal to the first interphalangeal crease, or the area between the proximal digital crease and the M.P. point. Much less frequently, a nodule may be found in the palm, proximal to the inferior palmar crease, between the skin and aponeurosis. Its adhesion to the aponeurosis is only secondary and comes from intimate contact with that structure.

When however, the disease attacks the aponeurosis, retractile bands are formed. These take their origin from the true aponeurosis and always follow a well defined course. We do not agree with Hueston when he says that they cannot be submitted to a rigid classification. The sclerotic process may selectively affect certain aponeurotic elements which we shall describe more fully later. Whether the lesions are found in frontal or sagittal, superficial or deep structures, the relations to the neurovascular elements are classical and anatomically predictable.

It is true that the proportions of the two types of lesions in one case may vary. There are essentially nodular forms, essentially retractile forms, and mixed forms with both nodules and retractile bands. Surgically the essential step is the excision of these bands which are responsible for flexion of the fingers. This excision is performed according to a technique based on the normal anatomy of the palmodigital aponeuroses.

This is why we think it is important to consider the anatomy of these structures. We studied these on the hands of adult corpses which we dissected with the utmost care. One of them happened to show Dupuytren's disease limited to the 5th finger. More than 50

colour photographs were taken at various stages of the dissection. The five figures shown in this article are drawings faithfully reproducing five of these photographs. They are neither compositions nor compound drawings. We have compared this study with our operative findings in more than 500 aponeurectomies.

1. ANATOMY OF THE MIDDLE PALMAR APONEUROSIS

By middle palmar aponeurosis is meant the central part of the superficial palmar aponeurosis, and excluding the aponeuroses of the thenar and hypothenar eminences. This middle palmar aponeurosis is triangular with the apex pointing proximally. It occupies the middle part of the palm between the two eminences. It is made up of two types of structures, the frontal and the sagittal.

The frontal plane (Figs. 2.1, 2.2) starts at the carpal annular ligament and is continuous with the terminal fibres of the palmaris brevis tendon. Proximally, it is narrow, dense and of uniform thickness. As it spreads out towards the root of the fingers, it gradually divides into four reinforced pretendinous strips. In the distal part of the palm, three frontal sheets with transverse fibres join the pretendinous strips, and close the angle of divergence of these strips. Their fibres, which constitute the superficial transverse ligament, are quite lax and run in a deeper plane than the vertical fibres of the pretendinous strips. Skoog stresses the point that the superficial transverse ligament is invariably spared in Dupuytren's disease, and we agree with this observation. The more proximal fibres of the superficial transverse ligament do not completely obliterate the angles of divergence of the pretendinous strips. In other words, these strips begin to diverge just proximal to the transverse fibres. There are triangular spaces filled by a more or less dense fatty tissue. These spaces with the sharp angle pointing proximally are limited laterally by the borders of the pretendinous strips, while their base is formed by the proximal border of the superficial transverse ligament.

The distal border of the superficial transverse ligament in the gaps between the pretendinous strips is always well defined. It forms the proximal border of a fatty zone which is lobulated, lax, slightly prominent and easily recognizable in the normal palm between the distal palmar crease, the axis of adjacent fingers and the commissures. In this fatty zone can be found the arteriovenous bifurcation and the two collateral nerves which more proximally were running under cover of the superficial transverse ligament.

In Fig. 1, the fatty lobules which have been left *in situ* between the index and middle fingers conceal the artery and the internal collateral nerve of the index.

Let us now consider the fate of the pretendinous strips

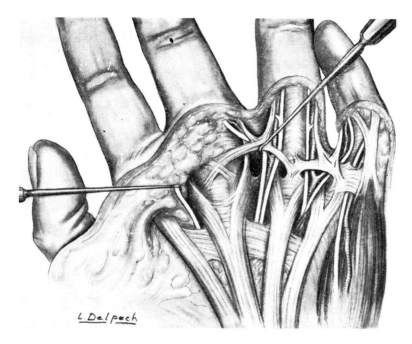

Figure 2.1
Palmar aponeurosis displayed after removal of skin and subcutaneous tissue. The pretendinous bands and their bifurcation as seen, the transverse superficial palmar ligament and the natatory ligament. Hooks retract the digital nerve and natatory ligament to show the course of the lateral and medial sheets to the middle finger.

distal to the superficial transverse ligament. This is mentioned in none of the anatomical descriptions that we found. In the classical diagrams, they are shown continuing down to the anterior aspect of the first phalanx. This, we think, is totally inaccurate. In fact, at the level of the metacarpal, the pretendinous strip divides V-wise into two strips which twist round, plunge inwards and run close to the lateral aspects of the capsule of the M.P. joint. A few transverse fibres come to form a small triangle, the apex directed proximally, which fills the angle between the strips.

No vertical fibres are found running in this angle. The

floor is formed by part of the fibrous sheath of the flexor tendons. More distally, opposite the base of the proximal phalanx, there is a complex, transverse aponeurotic structure, the interdigital palmar ligament, which we shall describe later. But there is one point on which we insist: the pretendinous strip, a palmar reinforcement of the superficial aponeurosis, does not continue longitudinally and in a frontal plane from the palm to the palmar aspect of the first phalanx. There is at the most a very loose, felty fibrous covering over the anterior aspect of the flexor sheaths. This lack of continuity in the fibres of the pretendinous strips is not generally known,

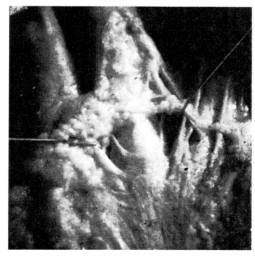

Figure 2.2
Photograph from which Figure 2.1 was drawn.

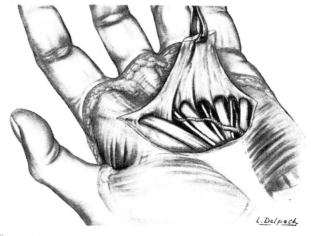

Figure 2.3
The palmar aponeurosis is being dissected from proximal to distal and the superior borders of the septa of Legueu and Juvara are placed under tension and the 7 canals can be clearly seen.

but Thomine has described it accurately. There does exist, as he states, an 'aponeurotic hiatus' between the termination of the pretendinous strip and the palmar interdigital ligament, opposite the metacarpal head. According to Thomine, the fibres of the pretendinous strip end by 'being inserted in the dermis'. We do not agree with this. They terminate in fact by plunging into the depth of the hand after bifurcating. This does not exclude the existence of a few tracts between the dermis and the aponeurosis, such as are present all over the palm and especially at the flexion creases. We shall later consider the anatomy of the aponeuroses in this palmo-digital junction zone.

Let us now come back to the middle palmar aponeurosis of which we have only described the frontal structures. From the deep surface of the palmar aponeurosis sagittal lamellae run vertically and separate the tendons from the neurovascular compartments of the palm (Figs. 2.3, 2.4, 2.5). These are the classical 'partitions'

of Legueu and Juvara, formed by so-called perforating fibres which run from the deep surface of the middle aponeurosis to the anterior surface of the deep aponeurosis, which itself joins the metarcapals and covers the interosseous muscles. These structures are clearly identifiable on a transverse section (Fig. 2.9) going through the middle palmar crease. First one recognizes the metacarpals with, stretched in a frontal plane between their anterior crests, the deep palmar aponeurosis. In a more anterior plane, the flexor tendons are seen running in the axis of the metacarpals. Between the flexor tendons, anterior to the intermeta-carpal space, the nerves have already divided, but not the digital arteries and veins which divide much more distally, very near the commissure. In a more superficial plane is the middle aponeurosis. The fibrous partitions are eight in all, one on either side of the tendon to each finger. On the section, one recognizes the seven compartments limited anteriorly by the plane of the palmar

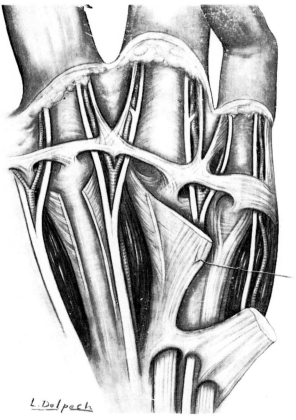

L. Delpech

Figure 2.4
The paratendinous septa of Legueu and Juvara have been divided on each side of the flexor tendons of the middle finger, so that the continuity of those septa with the lateral sheet of the finger is clearly seen. The important relation between the digital nerve and the fascia is shown with the lateral digital nerve to the middle finger passing anterior to this lateral digital sheet.

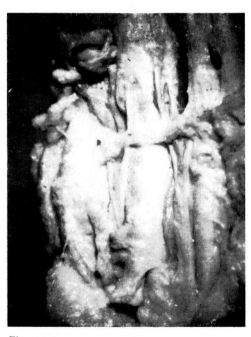

Figure 2.5
Photograph from which Figure 2.4 was drawn.

aponeurosis and laterally by the partitions of Legueu and Juvara. Four compartments transmit the tendons, and three transmit the neurovascular bundles and the lumbricals of the second, third and fourth interspaces. It will be noticed that the external neurovascular bundle of the index finger and the internal bundle of the 5th finger have no compartments of their own as they belong to the thenar and hypothenar regions respectively.

It is important to bear clearly in mind the inferior and superior borders of these partitions.

Proximally the falciform upper border begins well below the distal border of the annular ligament along a horizontal line which is about equidistant from the distal flexion crease of the wrist and the proximal digital crease. These partitions in fact never reach proximally beyond the superficial palmar arch and the tendinous origin of the lumbricals.

If the narrowed origin of the middle palmar aponeurosis is divided as proximally as possible, and if it is pulled down and freed from its connexions with the thenar and hypothenar aponeuroses, it is found that no deep attachments tie it down. Deep to it, one finds the superficial palmar arch and the division of the median nerve. Further down, folding of the middle palmar aponeurosis is restricted by the stretched sagittal partitions. The tendon and neurovascular compartments are exposed (Fig. 2.3). To lift the aponeurosis further, it then becomes necessary to divide the partitions down to their lower insertions. These insertions fuse with the pretendinous strips after their bifurcation on the lateral aspects of the capsules of the M.P. joints. We shall see later how the palmar aponeurosis, the interdigital palmar ligament and the digital aponeuroses become fused opposite the base of the first phalanx.

It is worth emphasizing the relationship of the tendons and the neurovascular bundles above and below the upper borders of the vertical intertendinous partitions.

Proximal to the origin of these septa the palmar aponeurosis forms a thick narrow sheet between the thenar and hypothenar eminences. The vessels and nerves are well superficial to the tendons so that when, at operation, this proximal segment of the aponeurosis is divided and the lateral margins freed, care is necessary to avoid the neurovascular bundles which completely conceal the flexor tendons. When the palmar aponeurosis is lifted the vessels tend to be lifted with it and, during the distal dissection, it is necessary to push them back to avoid injury in clearing the deep aspect of the aponeurosis.

More distally in the compartments between the septa the tendons diverge and the neurovascular bundles pass more deeply onto the same plane as the tendons.

2. THE DIGITAL APONEUROSES

The digital aponeuroses have been extensively studied over the years namely by Cleland (1878), Landsmeer (1949), Stack (1961), Thomine (1965). The most precise, the most complete and, to our mind, the most accurate is the description given by Thomine. Our observations differ from those of Thomine only in points of detail and our small disagreements are probably due to the fact that Thomine's studies are purely anatomical, while ours were influenced by our desire to explain the lesions observed in Dupuytren's disease and to contribute to surgical technique.

A very skilful dissector, Thomine studied simultaneously a number of thin sections of the foetal fingers and described extremely fine sheets which are not identified at surgical exploration. For this reason, we think they are of little practical importance. This difference is particularly striking when we consider the palmar neurovascular bundle in the finger. Thomine attaches much importance to these structures, and we do not deny that microscopy can reveal the presence of a superficial fibrous sheet in front of the bundle, as well as a deeper sheet, these two sheets joining within the bundle and around it, and forming a sheath which is elliptical in cross-section. We remember that at one time a similar sheath was described for the sterno-cleido-mastoid muscle and for the muscles surrounded by the middle cervical aponeurosis. For the benefit of surgeons, Cunéo produced a more simple description which stressed the planes of cleavage of the neck rather than the actual aponeuroses which a good anatomist can always separate into relatively artificial layers.

Personally, as we always found this vascular sheath a rather weak structure, in the normal and in the diseased hand, we shall consciously neglect it.

For another reason, we shall not mention Cleland's ligament, a frontal structure which is described as running between the skin and the lateral aspect of the phalanges, and is supposed to separate a dorsal from a palmar compartment. We have never succeeded in identifying this ligament which, according to Thomine, can only correspond to the artificial association of distinct tissue structures.

In the middle of the palmar aspect of the first phalanx, between the proximal digital crease and the middle crease, (proximal I.P. joint) we only found a lobulated fatty tissue with scattered fibrous partitions and no organized structure. In a deeper plane, there does exist a clear plane of cleavage between this fatty tissue and the anterior aspect of the fibrous tendon sheath. Is this enough to claim the existence of a digital sheath which limits the fatty layer on the one side and forms the deeper aspect of the neurovascular sheath on the other? We think not. In other words, we do not believe in the existence of a cylindrical fascial sheath for the whole length of the finger. It takes much skilful and tricky dissection to demonstrate the palmar part alone.

According to us, there is in the finger only one distinct aponeurotic structure which we shall describe under the name of lateral digital sheet. Our description will differ but little from Thomine's description of the lateral digital band. This band, which is most distinct at the level of the second phalanx, we regard as a lamellar structure in a larger sagittal sheet which is continued along the lateral aspects of the finger, from the commissure to the third phalanx. We think that our description is simpler, more succinct, and more likely to explain the relation between the anatomical structures and the pathological changes. Dissection of the lateral digital sheet is easy. One only has to remove the skin and then systematically to dissect out the fatty tissue. The lateral sheet is then exposed on the side of the finger, as can be seen from Fig. 6 which is an exact reproduction of a photograph. Horizontal sections made through the first phalanx and the proximal I.P. joint illustrate the description (Figs. 2.7, 2.8, 2.9).

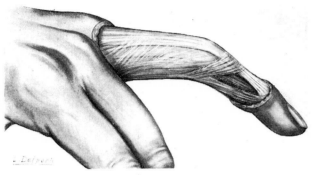

Figure 2.6
Medial fascia of middle finger showing retinacular ligament and band along the side of the middle phalanx, both hiding the neurovascular bundle.

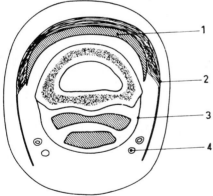

Figure 2.7
Transverse section through the proximal phalanx: (1) extensor apparatus; (2) lateral fascial sheet; (3) fibrous flexor sheath; (4) lateral digital nerve.

On the side of the proximal phalanx, it forms a sheet with a free anterior border, and a posterior border which bears a close relation to the extensor apparatus which, at this level, consists of the common extensor tendon plus the tendinous expansions of the interossei. Most of the fibres in this structure run vertical to the axis of the finger. Some run obliquely downwards and posteriorly to form a superficial strap over the extensor apparatus. Superficially, the skin over the lateral aspect of the finger opposite the sheet is thin and supple. At this level, there is but little fat, and very fine fibrous tracts tie the skin down to the sheet.

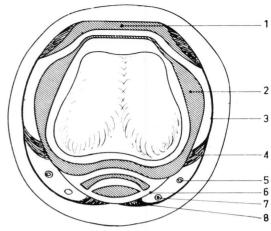

Figure 2.8
Transverse section of proximal interphalangeal joint: (1) extensor apparatus; (2) capsule and collateral ligament; (3) lateral fascial sheet; (4) expansion of lateral fascial sheet to capsule; (5) digital artery; (6) fibrous flexor tendon sheath; (7) digital nerve; (8) expansion of lateral fascial sheet to fibrous flexor sheath (origin of retinacular ligament).

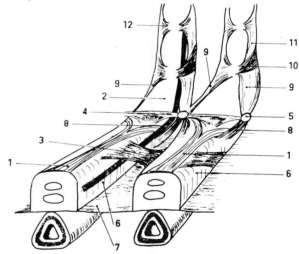

Figure 2.9
Diagram of fascial elements: (1) pretendinous band of palmar aponeurosis; (2) fibrous flexor sheath; (3) superficial transverse ligament of palm; (4) natatory ligament; (5) chiasma of natatory ligament; (6) septa of Legueu and Juvara; (7) deep transverse ligament; (8) origin of lateral digital fascial sheet, fusion of bifurcation of pretendinous band and distal extremity of septum of Legueu and Juvara; (9) lateral digital fascial sheet; (10) insertion of this sheet into the pulley of flexor sheath; (11) digital band at middle phalangeal level; (12) insertion of digital sheet on the pulley of the fibrous flexor sheath at distal interphalangeal level.

Finally, we note that this sheet has a uniform density along the distal three-quarters of the phalanx. Along the proximal quarter, at the origin of the sheet, near the commissure, the anterior border is markedly thicker than the posterior segment facing the extensor tendons. On a lateral view of the finger, the sheet completely conceals the neurovascular bundle which lies between the deep surface of the sheet and the anterolateral aspect of the flexor sheath. At this point, we must stress the close relation of the sheet to the nerve. Opposite the proximal phalanx, the sheet separates the lateral teguments from the neurovascular bundle. But a capital change occurs opposite the proximal interphalangeal joint. Fibres leave the sheet and find a strong insertion in the fibrous elements of the capsule of the joint. From the deep aspect of the sheet, fibres are given off which become imbricated with the lateral ligaments. From the anterior border, a bunch of fibres run across, and superficial to, the neurovascular bundle towards the middle of the flexor sheath where they find an insertion. On a face view of a dissected finger, the nerve, which is visible at the level of the proximal phalanx, is hidden opposite the I.P. joint by expansion of the sheet to the flexor sheath (Fig. 2.8). This expansion has been described by most authors, but some believe that it is inserted on to the bone. This, to us, seems impossible as, in a deeper plane, it could only reach the capsule laterally or the tendon sheath anteriorly. Being anterior, the insertion must be on the fibrous sheath. At that level, the neurovascular bundle does go through a tight fibrous tunnel formed posteriorly by the anterolateral aspect of the proximal I.P. joint and the flexor sheath, and anteriorly by the articular expansion of the lateral sheet. The slit is closed posteriorly by the capsular expansions of the sheet, and anteriorly, near the axis of the finger, by the expansion which crosses over the nerve and becomes closely adherent to the axis of the finger at the fibrous tendon sheath.

We now have to describe the lateral sheet opposite the 2nd phalanx, or in other words consider the fate of the fibres which have become inserted deep into the fibrous capsule of the proximal I.P. joint. The deeper ones, those which adhere to the capsule, run vertically along the side of the second phalanx and again become adherent to the lateral aspect of the next joint, i.e. the distal I.P. joint. There again there is a continuous strand of fibres which form a posterior cover for the extensor tendon. The density of this stand is quite different on the side of the finger and on its posterolateral aspect. On the side of the finger it forms a strong, solid band stretched between the lateral aspects of the I.P. joints like the string of a bow, the arc of which is formed by the concave border of the second phalanx. Thomine's description here is perfect in every way. There does exist a strand which joins the posterior border of the band to the border of the lateral strips given off by the extensor tendon. It is so thin, so tenuous that we can easily understand that it has been overlooked. But there are also more superficial fibres. They come off the anterior expansion of the strand which is adherent to the flexor sheath, opposite the

proximal I.P. joint; from there they run a distal and posterior course, the first ones running very posteriorly while the others run a more oblique course at about 45° to the axis of the phalanx—the whole structure forming a triangular sheet. Its summit lies anteriorly and is fixed to the fibrous sheath; it covers the lateral aspect of the second phalanx and, on the back of the same phalanx, it forms a strap which runs superficial to the extensor apparatus to which it is adherent. On the posterior aspect of the finger, the two triangular sheets meet in the midline after covering the medial and lateral aspects of the finger. These oblique fibres which strap the extensor tendon are stronger than those at the base of the first phalanx, though they occupy a comparable position. Although they belong to the lateral sheet, their oblique course makes them appear separate and they can be separated with a scalpel. In this way, the retinacular ligament of Landsmeer is artificially created. And having been thus created, it is assumed to have some physiological function which we think extremely doubtful. A number of authors have given confusing descriptions of this ligament; this comes out from the very summary diagrams which appear in a number of publications. In our figure, copied from a photograph, it appears as a distinct structure, as clearly as in the photograph published by our colleague Rabischong (Fig. 2.6).

3. THE PALMO-DIGITAL JUNCTION

What we are most interested in at this junction is the continuity between the palmar and digital structures, a continuity which can be demonstrated by deep dissection. It is because these palmodigital fibres lie deep on the sides of the metacarpophalangeal joints that the retractile fibrosis leads to the typical flexion deformities of Dupuytren's disease.

But before following these longitudinal fibres, we must consider in more detail the superficial, transverse palmar interdigital ligament which we have not yet described (Figs. 4 and 5).

Its fibres draw a long curve, slightly concave proximally, from the lateral border of the index finger to the medial border of the 5th finger. From its more superficial fibres, small fibrous strands run up to the dermis. As it crosses the base of each phalanx, its deep fibres become closely attached to the anterior aspect of the tendon sheath by a tough band. But these same deep fibres as they run across each commissural space, form an arch under which the neurovascular bundles run down to the fingers. At these arches there is an intricate mingling of fibres between the longitudinal fibres of the aponeurosis, the lateral digital sheet and the palmar interdigital ligament. As an example let us consider in detail this imbrication or 'chiasma', at the third interspace between the middle finger and the ring-finger (Figs. 2.10, 2.11). Opposite the neck of the third metacarpal, the medial branch of the bifurcated pretendinous thickening is twisted on its axis and runs deep into the hand. Its deep aspect is closely adherent to the capsule of the M.P. joint. The branch of the pre-tendinous thickening fuses with the inferior part of the partition of Legueu and Juvara. Together they run as a bundle of fibres under the transverse palmar ligament to form the medial laterodigital sheet of the middle finger. Thomine is quite right when he says that the superficial fibres of the transverse palmar ligament arising from the middle of the commissure,

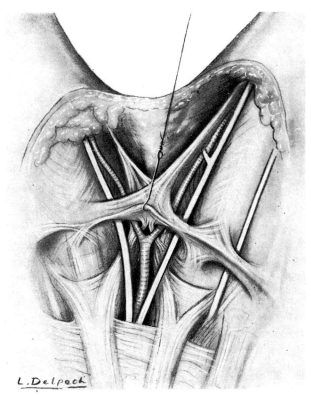

L.Delpech

Figure 2.10
In the web space the origin of the lateral fascial sheets of the finger and, crossing between the digital nerves and the aponeurosis, the chiasma of the natatory ligament.

become divergent distally, and run one branch towards the anterior border of the medial digital sheet of the middle finger, and the other to the anterior border of the lateral digital sheet of the ring finger. Thomine has suggested that the fibres running from the transverse palmar ligament to the lateral digital sheets are in fact the proximal origin of these sheets. We do not agree with this view and regard these fibres as an accessory structure. The true origin of the lateral digital sheets is constituted by the deep fibres which are the common continuation of the bifurcated pretendinous band and of the intertendinous partition of Legueu and Juvara.

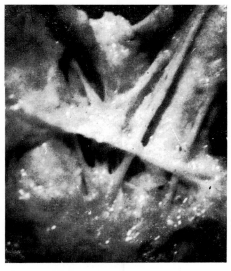

Figure 2.11
Photograph from which Figure 2.10 was drawn.

We must remember that they adhere closely to the capsule of the M.P. joint and are continuous with the anterior border of the deep aponeurosis. Although the anterior border of the digital sheet does give off a few fibres which mingle with the transverse palmar liga-ment, the majority of the fibres of the digital sheet run deep under the transverse palmar aponeurosis which have regrouped opposite the metacarpophalangeal joint.

At this level, it is essential that we describe accurately the relations of the nerves with the aponeurotic bands.

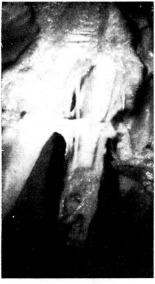

Figure 2.12
A clear demonstration of the digital nerve passing anterior to the aponeurotic expansion as it forms the proximal end of the lateral digital fascial sheet.

From a surgical standpoint, these relations are extremely important. If they are not clearly understood, aponeurectomy becomes a hazardous procedure.

On a transverse section of the hand, going through the distal third of the metacarpal, the sagittal partition can be seen lying between the tendons and the neurovascular bundle. Relative to the axis of the finger, the nerve is more peripheral than the partition. On a section of the finger at the level of the proximal phalanx, the digital sheet is more lateral than the nerve, again relative to the axis of the finger. These structures must have crossed at some point, and this point is in the line of the M.P. joint. The aponeurotic sheet after running longitudinally along the metacarpal, is deviated off the axis of the finger by the protruding metacarpal head. The lateral digital nerve crosses over it and continues along the side of the phalanx. More distally the divided branch of the digital artery follows a similar course. Figs. 2.10, 2.11, 2.12, especially 2.12, drawn from a specimen, show this crossing more accurately than any verbal description.

4. LESIONS AND MECHANISMS OF FLEXION IN DUPUYTREN'S DISEASE

We have said earlier that there are two types of lesions in Dupuytren's disease—the nodules and the bands.

The nodules superficially are very adherent to the skin, and deeply may become attached to the aponeurosis when this is present. But in a deeper layer, there is always a plane of cleavage between the nodule and the subjacent structure, provided this structure is not an aponeurosis. This is most obvious when a nodule is present in the midline, between the metacarpophalangeal crease and the neck of the proximal phalanx.

One usually has no difficulty in finding a plane of cleavage between the deep aspect of the nodule and the anterior aspect of the fibrous flexor sheath. But superficially, there usually exists a continuity between the nodule and the dermis. The nodule is always situated along a metacarpodigital axis. We agree with Hueston when he says that the nodule is formed in the fatty tissue, and at first develops independently of the aponeurosis. For the palmar nodules, this is still debatable. There is no palmar nodule without retractile sclerosis of the pretendinous aponeurotic band, and one is entitled to believe that the lesion started in the aponeurosis and later spread superficially to the subcutaneous fat and to the dermis. But at the level of the proximal phalanx, it is different: the nodule always lies on the midline where there is no recognizable aponeurotic structure. There the nodule develops in the subcutaneous cellular layer.

Proximally, every large mid-line phalangeal nodule is continued into a flattened, fibrous, ribbon-like strand towards the bifurcation of the pretendinous strip. More distally, the nodule is always adherent to the expansions of the lateral digital sheets which converge and become inserted in the midline, proximal to the tendon sheath insertion and to the proximal phalangophalangeal joint line (where the retinacular ligament finds its origin). It is at this level that excision of phalangeal nodules is most difficult and presents the risk of causing injury to the collateral nerve.

The nodules are usually what worry the patients most. In fact it is a relatively accessory lesion. The nodule does give rise to sclerosis and to cutaneous retraction, but it never leads to progressive flexion of the fingers. This flexion is due to the retraction of the aponeurotic structures forming bands, the situation of which depends on the anatomy of the aponeurosis.

This retractile sclerosis may be localized, or it might be extensive, or may be restricted to a palmar or a digital segment.

A large number of clinical forms can be distinguished. We shall only describe the most common ones.

(a) RETRACTION OF THE PRETENDINOUS PALMAR STRIPS

This can exist without nodule formation. In this case, adhesions to the skin are scanty: they are limited to a few millimetres here and there, proximal and distal to the point where the pretendinous strips cross the distal palmar crease. Such a lesion only results in flexion of the M.P. joint as, through its bifurcate insertion into the capsule of the M.P. joint, the shortened strip pulls on the base of proximal phalanx of the finger. The palmar skin is then often found to be thin and supple. In these cases, a simple subcutaneous fasciotomy will sometimes result in complete extension of the finger, which shows that metacarpophalangeal flexion comes exclusively from retraction of the pretendinous palmar strip. But in such cases, we usually restrict simple fasciotomy to old patients, female patients, rheumatic patients and patients in poor physical or mental health. We much prefer fasciectomy, but we only mention fasciotomy because it provides a good experimental demonstration of the pathogenesis of digital flexion in the pure palmar forms.

In the course of fasciectomies performed in the severe, purely palmar cases, affecting possibly two adjacent fingers, one may observe that the pathological process affects not only the pretendinous strip but also the intertendinous partition of Legueu and Juvara.

The latter is then found to be tough, thickened and difficult to cut with scissors. Sometimes, in its distal part, it ends as a cylindrical cord 2 to 3 millimetres across, which runs deep and is crossed over by the collateral nerve. Obviously the nerve must be dissected out before the cord is divided. It is easy to understand why a fasciectomy limited to the frontal fibres of the aponeurosis will be inadequate unless the excision is extended into the intermetacarpal space to include the strongest cord that pulls on the phalanx. This cord in fact constitutes the lower end of the partition of Legueu and Juvara after its fusion with the bifurcated branch of the pretendinous strip. In such a case, a single transverse incision across the pretendinous strip will hardly increase digital extension. In other quite common cases, one may find a combination of a palmar band (with or without palmar nodule) and a large prephalangeal midline nodule. Operation must then include palmar fasciectomy plus excision of the phalangeal nodule. As this nodule is attached proximally to the pretendinous strip and distally to the retinacular ligament of Landsmeer, it is easy to understand why it may lead to flexion of the middle phalanx relative to the proximal phalanx. Such flexion is never severe and usually yields readily after aponeurectomy and removal of the nodule. If it does not improve, there is usually something else: for example a diseased lateral digital sheet. In Dupuytren's disease it is this sclerotic and retractile lesion in the digital sheet which gives rise to the most severe forms, those which are included in group D of Michon and Tubiana.

(b) RETRACTION OF THE LATERAL DIGITAL SHEET

In the majority of cases, this retraction which leads to the formation of a lateral digital band is associated with a pretendinous palmar band. There are cases (relatively rare) where one finds a combination of palmar band, phalangeal nodule and lateral digital band. It is then difficult clinically to detect the lateral digital band before operation. One must always look for it at operation, and it will always be discovered when full extension is not restored by fasciectomy and removal of the phalangeal nodule. Quite often when there is a unilateral (on one side of the finger) or bilateral (both sides of the finger) digital band, there is also a palmar band but no phalangeal nodule. On palpation of the forcibly extended finger, the midline prephalangeal fatty tissue feels soft, yielding and normal. But on the sides of the finger one can feel a thin, taut cord which corresponds to the anterior border of the lateral digital sheet.

Surgically, one begins with the dissection, and the lifting of the palmar aponeurosis starting with its proximal end. This reveals a thickened, sclerosed, retracted pretendinous band which is not continuous on the palmar aspect with any abnormal tissue beyond the proximal digital crease. But it continues on the side of the metacarpal head and of the base of the proximal phalanx as a solid sheet which corresponds exactly to what we have described as the proximal attachment of the lateral digital sheet. But before coming to the latter, one must identify the nerve from the palmar side and follow it as it seems to emerge from the depths, and is crossed by the lateral prolongation of the pretendinous

strip. If the M.P. joint is in pronounced flexion, the anterior border of this band becomes superficial as it stretches from the palm to the side of the root of the finger. The band then lies at the same superficial level as the frontal plane of the palmar aponeurosis. It lifts the collateral nerve which is easily dissected out if one is aware of this pathological relation which, contrary to what has been claimed by some authors, does not represent an anatomical anomaly. Further away from the axis of the finger, the collateral artery crosses over the origin of the lateral sheet. Like the nerve it must be separated, identified, and treated with respect.

At this stage of the operation, there is no difficulty in dividing the lateral digital sheet at its origin, but the deeper fibres often escape the knife and are not easy to cut through as they lie trapped between the sides of adjacent M.P. joint. The surgeon then passes on to the finger where a Z-incision, with a midline vertical branch, is made on the proximal phalanx. We want to stress this point, as one is easily tempted into making a lateral or posterolateral phalangeal incision when faced with a lateral digital band. This type of incision which we have used ourselves on a number of occasions has little to recommend it. It gives a poor exposure of the distal portion of the digital band which is in the midline opposite the line of the proximal I.P. joint, at the origin of the retinacular ligament. It opens first on to the lateral band when in fact, before tackling this band, one must identify and protect the artery and nerve which are nearer the midline. Finally, the Z-plasty of the first phalanx has the immense and irreplaceable advantage of making possible closure of the palmar incision without tension and without a graft.

The edges of the Z are then raised. On the sides of the phalanx where the band runs, the lateral skin of the finger is very adherent to the sheet. The band must be freed right through to the lateral border of the interosseous tendon. But before going further, the nerve and collateral artery must be freed on the internal aspect of the lateral band (i.e. internal relative to the digital axis). Half way down the phalanx, this is easily done as the neurovascular bundle is perfectly free and is never included in a fibrous mesh. But it must then be followed right down to the proximal I.P. joint, it must be freed during its passage through the tunnel formed by the palmar expansion of the lateral sheet. Finding this tunnel and widening it must be done with great care and prudence.

The digital sheet has now been freed on two aspects. During the anatomical description, we said that its posterior border gave rise to fibres which form a covering for the extensor aponeurosis. This must now be divided vertically close to the border of the extensor apparatus. Further down the finger, opposite the proximal I.P. joint, one must also divide the band which bridges over the nerve and fuses in the midline with the

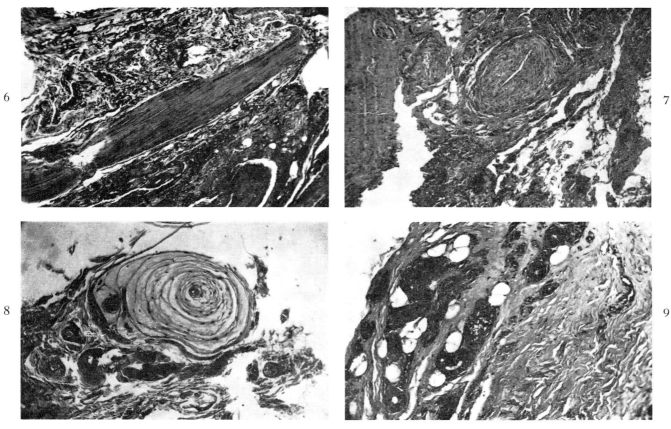

Figure 3.6
Shows absence of elastic fibres in the thickened aponeurosis and the abundance of areolar tissue (Wergert ×60).

Figure 3.8
A Pacinian corpuscle in the dermis (×100).

Figure 3.7
Thick walled arteries.

Figure 3.9
Deep dermal structure showing sweat glands adjacent to nodular thickening.

pathological changes, and we believe that the main lesions lie in the preformed connective tissue of the hand. The absence of elastic fibres in the pathological lesions seems to prove it.

Except in a small number of cases, we failed to demonstrate the presence of iron pigments. Unlike Skoog, we do not think that they are of any great significance or that they suggest micro-ruptures in the fibres.

On the whole, we can conclude that the contribution of histology in Dupuytren's disease is extremely disappointing. It does little else than confirm what was suspected clinically and observed at operation, namely the presence of *fibrosis*. It gives no clues as to the starting

point of the fibrosis, its histogenesis and its aetiology. long time. But it is difficult to agree entirely with Hueston's theory which claims that Dupuytren's disease is primarily a disease of prefascial adipose tissue which later extends to the palmar aponeurosis.

In our opinion, the hypervascularization, the venous stasis, and the presence of collections of round cells represent a reaction of the tissues rather than the initial

The more interesting observations are probably the absence of an inflammatory reaction, the absence of metamorphic changes in the ground substance, and the rarity of pigment deposits. These negative observations neither prove nor disprove existing aetiological theories.

REFERENCES

NEZELOF, C. & TUBIANA, R. (1958). La maladie de Dupuytren. Étude histologique. *Semaine des Hôpitaux de Paris,* **34** (18), 1102.

4. AETIOLOGICAL QUESTIONS IN DUPUYTREN'S CONTRACTURE

John T. Hueston

It is because of the tantalizing nature of this pathological condition known as Dupuytren's contracture that it receives so much attention. Students of this condition all feel that the solution to the enigma of Dupuytren's contracture must lie just around the next corner—but as each corner is turned we find yet another ahead of us.

Despite an enormous amount of study the cause of Dupuytren's contracture remains unknown—even the nature of the condition is still uncertain—and general agreement has not yet even been reached as to the primary focus of origin in as confined a space as the palm of the hand.

Only by the collection of data both clinical and histological and a regular reviewing and discussion of the uncertain aspects of this condition can we hope to turn the ultimate corner together.

In presenting this review of the aetiological researches my aim is not only to try to clarify the present position but to ask some questions which need to be answered—and thus perhaps to play the role of 'agent provocateur'.

It is human nature that each new generation of surgeons will question many of the attitudes and opinions of the previous generation and it is not only hoped but expected that our continuing questioning of this specific disease will provoke further research in the next decades both by checking on previous studies and promoting new ideas.

AETIOLOGICAL QUESTIONS

Our continuing search for the nature of Dupuytren's contracture is most conveniently directed by asking:
Who gets it?
What course does it run?
What therapy influences it?
What is its structure?
What is its mechanism of production?
Finally then, can it be prevented?
Only the contributions of the past few years can be reviewed in this paper but an attempt to assess the problem up to that point has already been published (Hueston, 1963).

WHO GETS IT?

A major problem exists when attempts are made to compare statistics relating to Dupuytren's contracture in different countries. Definitive population studies by the same observer in different racial groups are needed to confirm the growing impression that the incidence and perhaps even the nature of Dupuytren's contracture differs greatly over the continent of Europe.

Dupuytren's contracture is a European disease, being so rarely seen in non-Caucasian races as to make suspect the purity of racial descent of any such individual afflicted. However, the high incidence reported by Thieme (1968) in Scotland had only been approached in Europe by previous studies from Scandinavia, Wales and England (Early, 1962).

The high incidence found personally in Melbourne is closely related to that in Edinburgh and reflects the early colonization of Australia by the Scottish, English and Irish—producing a distillation of 'Dupuytren's families' in this country.

No comparable studies are available from eastern Europe but the magnitude of surgical intervention advocated by Dabrowski (1967) suggests a lack of familiarity with large numbers of patients with this condition. The Mediterranean races have an even lower incidence if the smaller surgical series reported from these countries are any indication.

In Edinburgh, Thieme (1968) has extended the genetic studies of Ling (1963) who found that 60 per cent of first degree age-weighted relatives had Dupuytren's contracture compared with 25 per cent of the general population. He had also confirmed the higher incidence in epileptics (36·9 per cent) compared with 25 per cent in the general population. Indeed he found Dupuytren's contracture to be 15 times commoner in epileptics than in the general population—disproving in the same epileptic study that prolonged administration of barbiturates is associated with a higher incidence of Dupuytren's contracture.

Therefore Dupuytren's contracture appears to be inherited as a dominant gene and, as idiopathic epilepsy is also accepted as being genetically determined, it would appear that some linkage from adjacent genes may explain the frequent coincidence of Dupuytren's contracture in epilepsy in the same person (James, 1968).

With a varying incidence of the gene and a varying penetrance in individuals it is clear that statistics on the natural history and indeed on the surgical results may be predetermined to be different from one racial group to another. For instance Gosset (1970) has found that patients with a strong diathesis and showing ectopic lesions such as knuckle pads and plantar lesions are rare in France. Such a national difference does not appear to be operating when the long term assessment of results in Austria (Millesi, 1966), match those in England (Hakstian, 1966) but it should be borne in mind as a possible cause of otherwise conflicting views on this disease. In other words there may be different racial patterns of Dupuytren's contracture as well as different racial incidences.

NATURAL HISTORY

The difficulty of dating the onset of Dupuytren's contracture is most readily shown by asking a patient who is requesting treatment for one hand if the other hand is involved. Often a definite early lesion is present without the patient being aware of it. Likewise the precise details of progression are often only vaguely remembered, but it is generally accepted that phasic progression is common. An attempt to account pathologically for this phasic course has been proposed by Millesi (1966) who has also provided the first long-term follow-up of untreated patients and has shown in general an increased rate of activity in the first 4 years and in the more severely deformed cases. The effect of a stronger disposition or Dupuytren's diathesis is well recognized, where associated lesions such as knuckle

pads, plantar lesions, forearm lesions, (Boyes, 1968) and even gingival lesions and tendo Achilles (Hueston, 1971) may occur.

The importance of recognizing not only the general nature of the disease predisposition, but also the life-long progression in most cases is best seen in relation to the assessment of results of therapy. While the majority of recurrences occur within 1 or 2 years after fasciectomy (Hueston, 1962; Tubiana, 1967) and may reflect a virtually 'post-traumatic' effect in the remaining palmar tissues, Hakstian and Millesi have shown a continuing incidence of recurrence over 10 and 12 years. This is consistent with the natural progress of the disease already demonstrated. It would seem that, particularly in strongly predisposed individuals, we are unable to influence by surgery the activity rate in un-operated areas, except perhaps to increase it.

EFFECT OF THERAPY

Conservative treatment has not yet been shown to have any effect on the natural history of Dupuytren's contracture (Hassler, 1967).

Gonzalez (1967), however, has shown that involution can follow simple division of the deforming band—nodule mechanism even in young active lesions provided that renunion of the divided structures is prevented by interposing a full thickness skin graft in the incisional defect (Figs. 4.1, 4.2). Fasciotomy has always enjoyed a

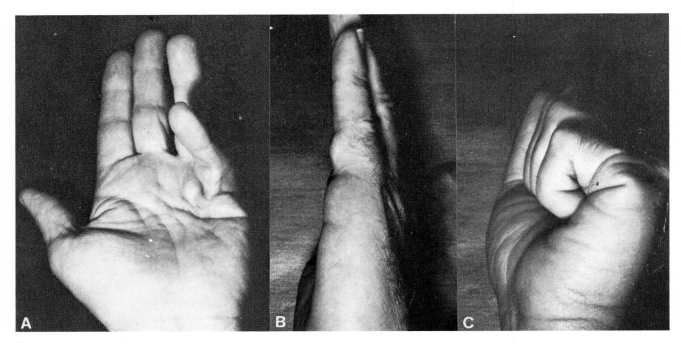

Figure 4.1
Open fasciotomy and Wolfe graft showing (A), preoperative deformity; and (B, C), the result with retained correction 2 years later. (Patient of Dr. R. Gonzalez).

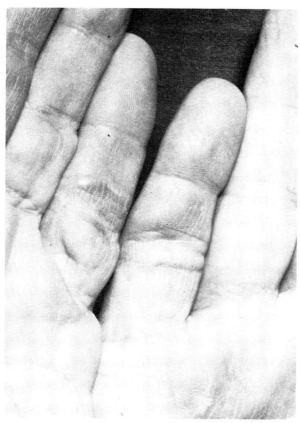

Figure 4.2
The result 2 years after an open fasciotomy and Wolfe graft on both little fingers of the same patient as shown in Figure 4.1, treated by Dr. R. Gonzalez.

definite place in the treatment of Dupuytren's contracture and, in elderly patients with discrete bands, is often seen to be followed by complete atrophy of these virtually inactive fibrous structures. The involution of active nodules seen after the Gonzalez procedure raises the question of the traction-tension factor in aetiology expounded by Luck (1959).

An even more exotic approach is the enzymic fasciotomy of Bassot (1964, 1968). By the injection of proteolytic enzymes and spreading agents into the deforming band-nodule mechanism, it is possible to weaken the band sufficiently to allow its passive rupture without resort to incisional surgery (Fig. 4.3). Bassot like Gonzalez has noted atrophy of the local fibroblastic nodules following this release of longitudinal tension. The long term results of these 'open' and 'closed' fasciotomies are awaited with interest as they could provide aetiological information relating to the subsequent behaviour of Dupuytren's contracture tissue left otherwise undisturbed in the palm and digits.

These late results could be compared with the results of fasciectomy where the skin has been surgically disturbed and either reapplied or replaced.

Recurrence after standard procedures of limited or radical fasciectomy are almost equal in the digits although Millesi (1966) has reduced palmar recurrences to 7·7 per cent by an extensive aponeurosectomy.

It is the digital recurrence which is more important functionally and aetiologically and which is the object of increasing study. In this regard two factors deserve study. The fibrous structures of the digit may be more difficult to extirpate than those of the palm and hence

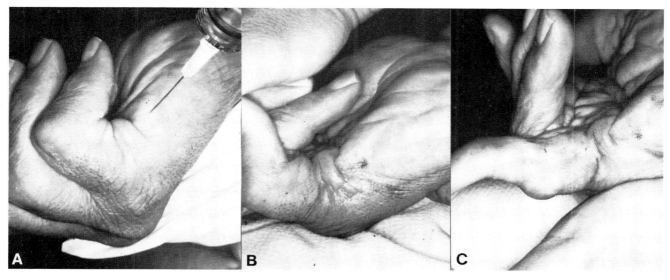

Figure 4.3
The right little finger is severely flexed at more than right angles at both MP and PIP joints in this elderly emphysematous patient, regarded by the anaesthetist as too ill even for regional anaesthesia! A, injection of Trypsin; B, 15 minutes after injection of Trypsin it is possible to begin to rupture the contracted fascial bands, and C, to correct the metacarpophalangeal joint completely and the proximal interphalangeal joint considerably.

may remain as foci for recurrence; the detailed anatomical studies of Stack (1973) and Gosset (1966) being relevant here. Also the circulatory control of the finger may be different from that of the palm and thus may be related to the higher digital recurrence rate, in view of the observation that skin graft replacement of the digital skin prevents local recurrence (Hueston, 1969) This concept makes it necessary not only to study the fibrous structures of the hand but also their overlying tissues if the aetiology is to be unravelled. Studies of the role of the dermis in the neurovascular control of the volar integument of the hand and fingers may bring us closer to the basic mechanism of production of Dupuytren's contracture.

The involution of Dupuytren's contracture tissue when transplanted from the palm (Fig. 4.4) despite retaining its attached dermis, may be related either to

hand and in some way as initiating the production of nodules over the surface of the remaining aponeurosis. Local injury can produce the same effect (Kauffmann and Straub, 1968; Hueston, 1968) although it is noted that, when a foreign body is found in relation to Dupuytren's contracture at operation it is not necessarily within the centre of the proliferating nodule. The local factors controlling fibroplasia require further study.

STRUCTURAL CHANGES

It is most likely that, as in most conditions, the basic tissue elements of the palm in Dupuytren's contracture are normal but are behaving in an abnormal manner under the influence of predisposing local and general factors. A report (Skoog, 1948) that the major bands in collagen fibrils from Dupuytren's contracture were

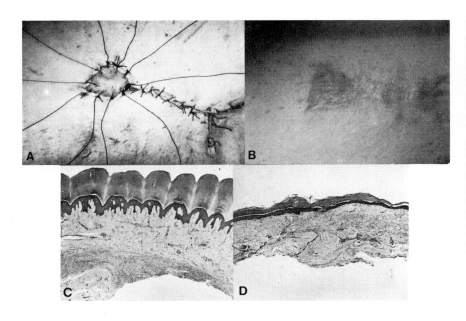

Figure 4.4
A free graft of palmar skin infiltrated with Dupuytren's tissue taken from the volar aspect of the base of the little finger which had been subjected to Wolfe graft replacement. The palmar skin has been switched to the donor site in the upper arm from where the Wolfe graft had been taken for the finger. Six months later the histology of the palmar skin has changed from the infiltrated thick highly keratinized skin to an almost papery scar-like pattern resembling more that of the upper arm and showing no evidence of residual Dupuytren's contracture within the dermis of the transplanted palmar skin.

loss of traction forces, and may thus be consistent with the fasciotomy effect of Gonzalez and Bassot; or it may reflect an alteration in the function of the presumably denervated dermis transplanted with it; or it may be a failure to respond by the new bed of subcutaneous fat of the upper arm with which the abnormal tissue has been brought into contact. Further study of this phenomenon is of aetiological importance.

Extension in unoperated areas of the hand has been seen to appear after limited fasciectomy even within the first postoperative month. The aetiological significance of this phenomenon cannot be ignored as it indicates a mechanism of local origin which is capable of acting while the hand is virtually at rest. The operative intervention must be viewed as a local injury to part of the

closer together than the usual 640 Ångstrom repeating period of native collagen was not confirmed by Peacock (1964).

The hyperplastic nodule is an essential structural component of Dupuytren's contracture because it must be the site of origin of the contracting force. Collagen does not contract under physiological conditions and the forces produced within the tissue of Dupuytren's contracture must be the result of cellular activity within the hyperplastic areas.

The anatomical studies of Thomine in this volume draw attention to the relative paucity of normal fascial structures in the very regions where Dupuytren's contracture is most common, namely in the distal palm and in the middle of the proximal segment of each finger.

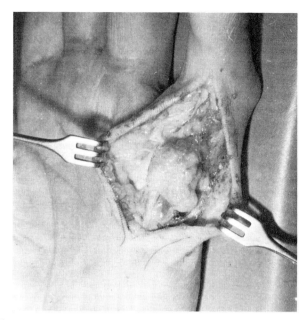

Figure 4.5
Surgical exposure of a palmar nodule showing its situation anterior to the plane of the palmar aponeurosis.

He suggests that an extrafascial explanation for the production of this new fibroplastic tissue should be sought. Perhaps metaplasia is the answer we seek?

Histological studies by Dabrowski (1967,a) confirm the plane of the hyperplastic nodules to be on the anterior surface of the palmar aponeurosis. The deep aspect is well known to remain free of nodular formation and the subaponeurotic fat to remain free of infiltration. That the transverse fibres of the aponeurosis usually remain clear of involvement has prompted Skoog (1967) to leave these behind at fasciectomy. These transverse fibres become tense when full finger flexion is forced and the aetiological implication is clear that, conversely, longitudinal traction may be a factor in determining the distribution of the longitudinal bands—although their more superficial situation and intimate connections to the structurally complex dermis may play as great a role.

The frequently bizarre arrangement of closely juxtaposed mature collagen fibres with extremely cellular areas within a palmar nodule is a distinct feature of the histological structure of Dupuytren's contracture.

An attempt to explain this on serial cellular destructions of the locally altered collagen (Fig. 4.6A) was made by Millesi (1966) who claims to be able to tell the age of the pathological change from the histological picture. While this may need confirmation it drawn attention to the intimate relation of fibrous and cellular elements.

The macroscopic observation of a hypercellular nodule superficially applied to a raised tight and shortened longitudinal band (Fig. 4.5) raises the possibility that the longitudinal fibres have been drawn up into the nodule by the cellular action therein (Fig. 4.6B). The analogy between applying the flat of the hand onto a handkerchief and then gradually crumpling up the handkerchief into the palm by the action of the fingers (Fig. 4.7) may be used to illustrate a possible means of production of juxtaposed collagen bands and hypercellular areas. Sections show abrupt cessation of longitudinal fibres at the band margin but these may be demonstrating only the newer collagen fibres laid down under the influence of work hypertrophy as the longitudinal traction forces are built up. These added fibres would be expected to be the first to resolve and disappear on release of the longitudinal tension which follows fasciotomy.

The relative uniformity of the histological picture in knuckle pads and plantar lesions, without so much mixture of collagen bands seen in palmar digital lesions may be correlated with the absence of anatomical contracture in these ectopic sites. Three-dimensional reconstructions of contracting and non-contracting nodules are required to elucidate this fundamental aspect of the contracture process in Dupuytren's contracture.

While the hyperplastic nodule is the essential structural element of Dupuytren's contracture, its precise site of origin is not perfectly clear. A study of the margin of such a nodule where it is passing into the adjacent tissue of the palm often shows a progressive replacement of fat by fibrous septa whose cells are clearly arising from the perivascular cellular cuff of the prolific vascular plexus of the palm. It will require precise demonstration and measurement of the vascular pattern of the normal palm and of the palmar tissue in Dupuytren's contracture to be certain if the vascular bed is actually increased.

It has certainly not been possible to verify the claim of Davis (1965) that there is an abnormality of the ulnar artery in every hand of Dupuytren's contracture. Any definitive demonstration of vascular bed abnormality will then need to be reappraised to determine whether this variation is primary or secondary, in the mechanism of production of the Dupuytren's tissue. Almost certainly it will be secondary, providing an essential step in the pathological process. Whatever is then found to be responsible for the anatomical or physiological vascular bed abnormality will then be the cause of Dupuytren's contracture.

MECHANISM OF PRODUCTION

The normal palmar aponeurosis is quite sparse and not easy to fix for systematic histological study. On the

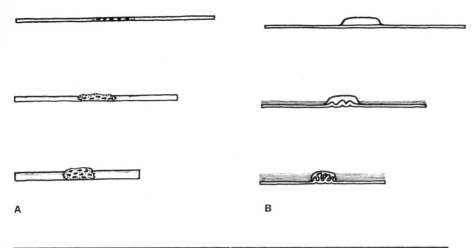

Figure 4.6
Diagram of the two main theories of the pathogenesis of Dupuytren's contracture: A, intrinsic theory—changes within the normal pre-existing palmar aponeurotic fibres lead to the formation of hyper-cellular nodules and hypertrophic bands; B, extrinsic theory—tissue overlying the anterior aspect of the palmar aponeurotic structure, between the aponeurosis and the dermis, produce a shortening of the aponeurotic structures by second-ary involvement of these structures and the development of bands by work hypertrophy secondary to the tension produced within them.

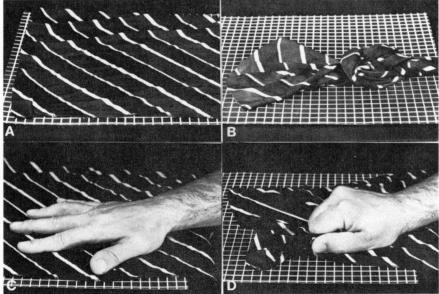

Figure 4.7
To demonstrate the intrinsic and extrinsic theories of Dupuytren's contracture. A, B, shortening is produced by the tissues literally becoming contracted into a knot; C, D, the tissues become shortened by application of an external focus applied to them and inducing shortening.

other hand the massive bulk of some specimens from Dupuytren's contracture indicates the considerable degree of hyperplasia which has occurred. Does this all arise within the scanty palmar aponeurosis or is it a more regional change throughout a block of palmar tissue? The palmar aponeurosis and other normal fibrous structures of the palm certainly are involved early in this process with the production of skin pits and joint flexion. The ultimate force generated in the process is such as to shorten the normal anatomical fibrous framework up to half its length (Fig. 4.8); since force requires energy and energy can only come from living cells, it is clear that the cellular areas are the fundamental source of the contracture in Dupuytren's contracture.

The secondary changes in and around the normal fibrous structures of the palm may overshadow the primary phenomenon of hyperplasia. These are the production of more and thicker collagen fibres arranged longitudinally or obliquely in the line of the contracting force. The originally fine palmar aponeurosis strands have had added to them such masses of new similarly arranged fibrous tissue that they often exceed the bulk of a flexor tendon. This addition of fibrous tissue is mainly on the anterior aspect of the pretendinous aponeurotic band and throughout its normal plane but never onto its deeper aspect. Work hypertrophy must be the major factor in this band production—secondary to the nodules—as Luck (1959) has already suggested. The rapid atrophy of these thickened bands after fasciotomy supports this concept. Such a super-ficial addition of the newer fibrous elements is consistent with the new forces arising on the superficial aspect of the pretendinous band from the fibroplasia in the subcutaneous palmar space. The more deeply placed transverse aponeurotic fibres are less accessible and it could be argued that in them the stretching force is limited by the flexor muscle power whereas finger extension is often by more powerful exogenous forces with more obvious resultant band production.

If there is an increase in local vascularity of the palmar tissues it is not yet possible to say if this precedes or

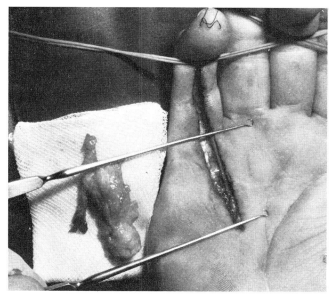

Figure 4.8
Comparison of the length of the operative incision and the length of the tissue excised demonstrates the great degree of shortening of the pre-existing tissues within the finger in Dupuytren's contracture.

follows the other structural changes but, in view of the association of Dupuytren's contracture with alcoholism, invalidism and local disuse, it is probable that a vascular—or at least a vasomotor change plays an important role in the pathogenesis of this condition.

If local trauma, surgical or accidental, can induce a rapid production of new lesions nearby, the possibility of a mechanism of local vasomotor changes seems worthy of further study. Presumably the perivascular proliferation is associated with this alteration in behaviour of the local vascular bed, and certainly the fibroplasia is related to the local vascular pattern. Because a diversity of agencies can produce the same basic sequence of local pathological changes it suggests strongly that some local form of final common pathway exists in the mechanism of the pathogenesis of Dupuytren's contracture.

The age of the patient has an influence on the effect of this local mechanism. An association with specific injury is more commonly seen in younger patients (Hueston, 1969) this age distribution (Fig. 4.9) closely resembles that seen in patients producing recurrence

(Hueston, 1963). On the other hand the trauma of fasciotomy, or a traumatic rupture of a band in an elderly patient almost invariably leads to disappearance of the band, as distinct from this tendency to a flareup of local activity in the younger age groups.

The hypothesis that there is a neurovascular basis for this abnormal tissue behaviour in the subcutaneous palmar space was first proposed by Abbe (1888) and

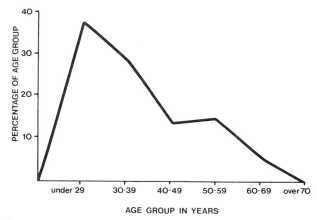

Figure 4.9
The age distribution of 58 patients in whom the clinical onset or aggravation of Dupuytren's contracture was personally observed within only a few months after a specific injury or regional injury to the limb. The highest incidence is seen in the younger age groups (reproduced by permission of the Editor, *Medical Journal of Australia*).

has been supported more recently by Nezelof and Tubiana (1958), Clarkson (1961), Hueston (1963), Kvicala (1963), and Dabrowski (1967b).

Such a hypothesis provides a possible explanation for the production of a similar pathological process in the palm by a diversity of local and general factors. The role of the dermis in this neurovascular theory could well be by the provision of a mediating neurovascular organ.

Recurrence can occur in predisposed patients with a strong Dupuytren's diathesis when the local skin is replaced after fasciectomy. No recurrence occurs if this local skin is removed and replaced by a free graft of skin from elsewhere (Hueston, 1969).

The skin of mammals has an inverse relationship between the number of hair follicles and the number of specialized nerve endings (Winkelmann, 1960). The fate of these elements after grafting requires further study. The nerve endings in grafted human skin and therefore the function of the grafted skin are not the same as in the normal palmar skin. Moreover a free graft is at first totally denervated and some of the specific cutaneous nerve endings may totally disappear. On reinnervation it is unlikely that absolutely normal neural integrity will be re-established. Studies are at present in progress to try to identify the differences between the neuroanatomy of normal palmar skin and of re-innervated Wolfe grafts. If some functional neural element is constantly lacking then it may indicate a means by which the underlying tissue is freed of the potential to form Dupuytren's contracture. A similar physiological study of local cutaneous reflex mechanisms would be of great interest and relevance.

In the subcutaneous plane, particularly along the line of the digital nerves, Pacinian corpuscles can at times be so large as to be a nuisance in defining the neurovascular bundles during fasciectomy, and an aetiological relationship—perhaps playing a role in the local vasomotor reflex control of fibroplasia—obviously suggests itself. However, a limited study of 10 hands in cadavers over 65 years of age showed Pacinian corpuscles equally abundant in the same distribution and up to 7 mm in length.

A more physiological study into the possible role of the Pacinian corpuscles is warranted.

In conclusion, while some local recurrences may be due to retained Dupuytren's tissue infiltration within the replaced dermis this does not apply to all cases and it is very likely that the dermis, being a complex organ, normally plays an important role in controlling the state of the subcutaneous tissue immediately related to it. Detailed study of this role of the dermis in the hand is essential, particularly within the subcutaneous palmar space where the dermis is intimately bound down by fibrous strands to the aponeurotic layer, if we are ever to arrive at a complete understanding of the mechanism of production of Dupuytren's contracture.

REFERENCES

ABBE, R. (1888). Dupuytren's finger contraction. *Medical Record (New York),* **33,** 237.

BASSOT, J. (1965). Traitement de la maladie de Dupuytren par exérèse pharmacodynamique isolée ou complétée par un temps plastique uniquement cutané. *Lille chirugical,* **20,** 1.

BASSOT, J. (1969). Traitement de la maladie de Dupuytren par exérèse pharmacodynamique. Bases physio-biologiques. Techniques. *Gazette des Hôpitaux de Paris,* 557.

BOYES, J. H. & JONES, F. E. (1968). Dupuytren's disease involving the volar aspect of the wrist. *Plastic and Reconstructive Surgery,* **41,** 204.

CLARKSON, P. (1961). The aetiology of Dupuytren's contracture. *Guy's Hospital Reports,* **110,** 52.

CLARKSON, P. (1966). *Contractures of the Fingers in Clinical Surgery* (edited by Robb and Smith). London: Butterworth.

DABROWSKI, T. (1967). Microscopic lesions in Dupuytren's disease. *Acta medica polonica,* **8a,** 477.

DAVIS, J. E. (1965). On surgery of Dupuytren's contracture. *Plastic and Reconstructive Surgery,* **36,** 277.

EARLY, P. (1962). Population studies in Dupuytren's contracture. *Journal of Bone and Joint Surgery,* **44B,** 602.

GONZALEZ, R. (1967). In: *Current Practice in Orthopaedic Surgery,* vol. 4, p. 175. St Louis: Mosby.

GOSSET, J. (1966). Anatomie des aponévroses palmo-digitales. In: *Maladie de Dupuytren.* Paris: Expansion Scientifique Française.

HAKSTIAN, R. W. (1966). Resultats eloignes de l'aponévrectomie étundu. In: *Maladie de Dupuytren.* Paris: Expansion Scientifique Française.

HUESTON, J. T. (1962). Digital Wolfe grafts in recurrent Dupuytren's contracture. *Plastic and Reconstructive Surgery.* **29b,** 342.

HUESTON, J. T. (1963). *Dupuytren's Contracture.* Edinburgh: Livingstone.

HUESTON, J. T. (1968). Dupuytren's contracture and specific injury. *Medical Journal of Australia,* **1,** 1084.

HUESTON, J. T. (1969). The control of recurrent Dupuytren's contracture by skin replacement. *British Journal of Plastic Surgery,* **22,** 152.

JAMES, J. I. P. (1968). Paper presented to British Hand Club, East Grinstead Meeting.

KAUFFMANN, M. S. & STRAUB, L. R. (1968). Dupuytren's contracture and the relationship of trauma, presented to the American Society for Surgery of the Hand.

KVIVALA, V., ODVARKOVA, J., SEDLACEK, J. & VACEK, J. (1963). Neurogenic etiology of Dupuytren's contracture. *Acta chirurgica plastica,* **5,** 227.

LING, R. S. M. (1963). The genetic factor in Dupuytren's disease. *Journal of Bone and Joint Surgery,* **45B,** 709.

LUCK, J. V. (1959). Dupuytren's contracture: a new concept of the pathogenesis correlated with surgical management. *Journal of Bone and Joint Surgery,* **41A,** 635.

MILLESI, H. (1966). Evolution clinique et morphologique de la maladie de Dupuytren. In: *Maladie de Dupuytren.* Paris: Expansion Scientifique Française.   H

NEZELOF, C. & TUBIANA, R. (1958). La maladie de Dupuytren. Étude histologique. *Semaine des Hôpitaux de Paris,* **34,** 1102.

PEACOCK, E. E. (1964). Dupuytren's contracture. In: *Reconstructive and Plastic Surgery* (edited by J. M. Converse), vol. 2, p. 1728. Philadelphia: Saunders.

SKOOG, T. (1948). Dupuytren's contracture. *Acta chirurgica scandinavica,* **96,** suppl. 139.

SKOOG, T. (1967). The superficial transverse fibres of the palmar aponeurosis and their significance in Dupuytren's contracture. *Surgical Clinics of North America,* **47,** 443.

STACK, H. G. (1973). *The Palmar Fascia.* Edinburgh: Churchill Livingstone.

THIEME, W. T. (1968). Personal communication.

TUBIANA, R. (1969). Les conceptions actuelles du traitement chirurgical de la maladie de Dupuytren. In: *Orthopédie et Traumatologie, Conférences d'Enseignement,* 1967. Paris: Expansion Scientifique Française.

WINKELMANN, R. K. (1960). *Nerve Endings in Normal and Pathologic Skin.* Springfield, Ill.: Thomas.

5. THE GENETIC PATTERN OF DUPUYTREN'S CONTRACTURE AND IDIOPATHIC EPILEPSY

J. I. P. James

All who see Dupuytren's contracture frequently are aware that many patients know of other members of their family who have the same condition. In our series, as in many others, this is 10 per cent. Occasionally a patient is found with a knowledge of several generations with contracture. Such evidence, though needing confirmation is strikingly suggestive of an hereditary disease. In a disease as common as Dupuytren's contracture one must, however, be cautious in attributing this to a genetic effect when it could be explained by its great frequency in the population.

To study such a disease satisfactorily from the genetic standpoint it is necessary, therefore, to examine all the available relatives of a number of patients with Dupuytren's and to know the incidence in the general population.

In 1963 Ling published a paper on such an investigation. He took 50 patients from the Edinburgh Hand Clinic who had been diagnosed as having Dupuytren's contracture. From these he obtained knowledge of the whereabouts of their first, second and third degree relatives. Arrangements were made to visit these and a total of 832 relatives of the 50 patients were examined, entailing much travelling all over Britain.

Dupuytren's contracture is a peculiarly satisfactory disease to survey in this way. Examination of the hands and feet in the home without X-rays or investigation is adequate though there are, under such circumstances, a number of individuals in whom the changes are so slight that diagnosis is difficult. Such were rejected.

A major difficulty encountered in such surveys in a disease that has its onset in the later decades is that many individuals, relatives of the index case, will be too young to manifest Dupuytren's though they may later develop it. Duchenne-type muscular dystrophy and Huntington's chorea are two of several inherited diseases where the onset is delayed after birth. However, it is the children and younger adults who are easy to trace and easy to see.

Carter (1961) showed that if the average age at onset of a disease was known, a calculation was possible that allowed the young age of the relatives at the time of being seen to be taken into account. Whilst the age of onset of Dupuytren's is difficult to know and must be an approximation, Ling using 130 cases of his own and 656 from Early's (1962) survey was able to draw a curve of age of onset in men and women (Table 1, Fig. 5.1). From this it can be seen that a man of 45 has a 59 per cent chance of having Dupuytren's already if he is destined to develop it, a woman of the same age, only 17 per cent. When a man of 45 is seen in the study of relatives he is counted as 0.59 of an individual, a woman of the same age 0.17 of an individual. By this age-weighting of the relatives the probable true incidence can be estimated for a survey.

TABLE 1   Age of onset of Dupuytren's contracture in 786 patients (130 from present series and 656 from Early (1962)

Age in years	Male	Female
5–14	10	0
15–24	48	1
25–34	87	2
35–44	129	10
45–54	158	25
55–64	109	48
65–74	38	32
75–84	10	12
85–94	3	5
Unknown	39	20
Total	631	155

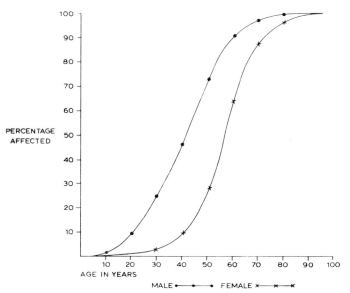

Figure 5.1

Population surveys are the other absolute require-ment in such family studies for it has to be shown that the disease is more common in these families than in the general population. I use 'general' advisedly because there will prove to be considerable differences when different countries are studied. It would seem probable that Dupuytren's does not occur among Negroes, Chinese and Asiatic Indians of pure stock, or if later cases become known, they will be exceptional since they are unknown at present to surgeons working amongst these races.

Several population surveys are available, the best by Early (1962) whose figures are shown (Table 2). They relate to the population of Bury, a town in Lancashire. Hueston (1960) carried out a smaller survey in the State of Victoria, Australia, and showed astonishingly high figures (Table 3), 25 per cent in males over 60 years of age. Ling, to amplify our knowledge in the elderly, examined 250 males and 250 females over 65 years of age in Edinburgh and showed a not dissimilar percentage

which increased to 28·5 per cent in very elderly males (Table 2). These two tables also compare the incidence of Dupuytren's in the families studied with these population surveys. They are not corrected for age-weighting. Even so the percentage affected in the families (Column 3) compared to the general population (Column 4, Table 2) is striking, in both males and females.

Let us return to the family studies. Amongst the 50 original cases, 8 or 16 per cent knew of other affected members of their family. Examination however, showed that 68 per cent of families had other affected members; in three other families there was strong hearsay evidence of contracture in deceased relatives or other relatives unavailable for examination because they lived outside Britain. Indeed the remaining families with no history of other cases apart from the original patient were either families with very young children or very small families with most relatives emigrants and unavailable.

Ling's findings in the relatives of these 50 patients

TABLE 2 Incidence of Dupuytren's contracture in the families studied, excluding propositi (columns 1, 2, 3, 6, 7 and 8) compared to the incidence in the general population in Lancashire (columns 4 and 9) (Early, 1962) and Edinburgh (columns 5 and 10)

	Male					Female				
	1	2	3	4	5	6	7	8	9	10
Age in years	Number examined	Number affected	Percentage affected	Percentage affected in general population	Percentage affected in Edinburgh geriatric survey	Number examined	Number affected	Percentage affected	Percentage affected in general population	Percentage affected in Edinburgh geriatric survey
0–14	98	1	1·02	—	—	90	0	—	—	—
15–24	75	3	4·0	0·1	—	52	0	—	—	—
25–34	51	5	9·8	0·2	—	57	2	3·5	—	—
35–44	48	8	16·7	1·2	—	64	4	5·5	—	—
45–54	56	8	14·3	4·1	—	59	3	5·1	0·5	—
55–64	42	11	26·2	10·1	—	46	9	19·5	1·4	—
65–74	24	17	70·8	14·1	25·6	33	8	26·2	6·2	17·8
75–84	14	9	64·3	18·1	28·9	17	10	58·8	9·0	17·0
85–94	—	—	—	—	28·5	6	3	50·0	—	17·0

TABLE 3 Incidence of Dupuytren's contracture in the families studied, excluding propositi (columns 1, 2, 3, 5, 6 and 7) compared to the incidence in the general population in Victoria, Australia (columns 4 and 8) (Hueston, 1960)

	Male				Female			
	1	2	3	4	5	6	7	8
Age in years	Number examined	Number affected	Percentage affected	Percentage affected in population of Victoria	Number examined	Number affected	Percentage affected	Percentage affected in population of Victoria
0–39	249	10	4·01	4·43	227	4	1·76	2·1
40–59	96	21	21·8	16·26	118	8	6·7	13·02
60 and over	58	31	53·4	25·29	82	27	32·9	20·39

TABLE 4   Incidence of Dupuytren's contracture in relatives of the propositi

Relationship	Total number examined	Weighted total (for age)	Number observed to be affected	Expected to be affected on single dominant hypothesis allowing for population incidence
Males				
First degree relatives				
Fathers	11	10·54	8	7·2
Brothers	56	39·47	21	27·1
Sons	25	3·32	1	2·28
Total first degree relatives	92	53·33	30	36·58
Second degree relatives				
Uncles	22	20·38	10	9·55
Nephews	83	13·76	5	6·43
Total second degree relatives	105	34·14	15	15·98
Third degree relatives				
First cousins	90	50·65	7	18·06
Females				
First degree relatives				
Mothers	13	9·98	7	6·86
Sisters	51	21·5	4	14·7
Daughters	31	1·452	0	0·99
Total first degree relatives	95	32·932	11	22·55
Second degree relatives				
Aunts	46	33·18	8	15·55
Nieces	77	2·557	2	1·19
Total second degree relatives	123	35·737	10	16·74
Third degree relatives				
First cousins	94	26·93	13	9·6

'age-weighted' for correction are seen in Table 4 compared to the expected number to be found with dominant inheritance. There is very satisfactory correlation between the age-corrected figures of the number of affected individuals observed and those theoretically expected if Dupuytren's were of dominant inheritance. The theoretical incidence is based on the hypothesis of dominance, fully expressed. The number in women under 75 is less than expected, the expression of the abnormal gene carrying Dupuytren's is delayed in women.

Two illustrative family trees from Ling's series are seen in Figures 5.2, 5.3.

In the family represented in Figure 3 it is probable that the trait was brought together by both the father and the mother in generation II and the siblings are homozygous for this abnormality; severe Dupuytren's occurred early in several of the family. It would seem possible that expression in homozygotes for this disease is earlier than average. Such individuals cannot be rare in so common a dominant inherited disease.

Whilst Ling's work proved the inheritance of Dupuytren's to be dominant the numbers were small and because of difficulty in seeing relatives in some families, minor discrepancies could be found by a critical study. It was, therefore, advisable to look at this problem in depth and Dr W. Thieme of Seattle working in Edinburgh on an N.I.H. grant reviewed the first degree relatives of 131 patients with Dupuytren's. He also

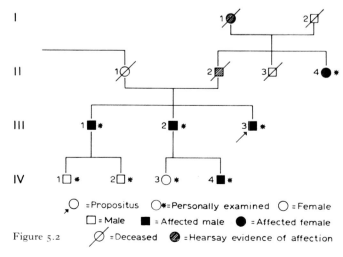

Figure 5.2

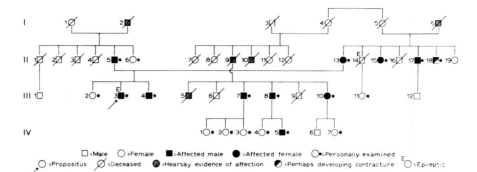

Figure 5.3

□ =Male   ○ =Female   ■ =Affected male   ● =Affected female   ○• =Personally examined
↗○ =Propositus   ∅ =Deceased   ◐ =Hearsay evidence of affection   ◑ =Perhaps developing contracture   ᴱ○ =Epileptic

studied the genetics of the Dupuytren–epilepsy association by investigating the latter disease in the Dupuytren's patients and their families and investigating the incidence of Dupuytren's in 88 patients with epilepsy from the Edinburgh Neurological Clinic and their first degree relatives.

Skoog (1948) first noted that epilepsy and Dupuytren's were seen frequently in the same patient, 42 per cent in an epileptic colony and in elderly epileptics it approached 90 per cent, Lund (1941), Skoog (1948). Early (1962), and Hueston (1963) found a high incidence, 4 to 5 per cent, of epilepsy in Dupuytren's patients, a finding any of us who have seen much of this disease would confirm. Thieme's findings are very interesting but as his results are unpublished I wish to do no more than summarize his findings and I am grateful for his permission to do so. Table 5 shows that epilepsy

The first degree relatives of the Dupuytren's totalled 492; after age weighting correction this gave 279 individuals. The expected population incidence of Dupuytren's in this number is 70, whereas 188 were observed to have Dupuytren's (Table 6). This is a 67 per cent incidence. Only a genetic factor could explain so high an incidence in such a chronic disease congregated in families. It is of course only one more confirmation of observations by many others. Burch

TABLE 6   Familial incidence compared to population incidence (Thieme)

| Number of 1st degree relatives | | Dupuytren's | | |
Seen	Corrected for age	Observed	Expected	P
492	279·0	188	70	< 0.01

TABLE 5   Observed association of Dupuytren's disease and epilepsy (Thieme)

Dupuytren's cases seen		Epilepsy found	Epilepsy expected	P
371		32 (8·6%)	1·86	< 0·001

Epileptic cases seen	Number corrected for age	Dupuytren's found	Dupuytren's expected	
111	66·7	32 (29%)	15·1	< 0·01

was several times more common in the 371 persons with Dupuytren's than expected by the population incidence. Similarly Dupuytren's was twice as common amongst the 111 epileptics.

(1966) has stated that Dupuytren's might be autosomal recessive inheritance, not autosomal dominant as suggested by Ling. Thieme (Table 7) showed the correlation of the observed incidence in the relatives

TABLE 7   A comparison of dominant and recessive modes of inheritance (Thieme)

Relationship	Total seen	Weighted total	Dupuytren's dominant hypothesis			Dupuytren's recessive hypothesis		
			Observed	Expected	P	Observed	Expected	P
Parent	47	38·4	32	22·9		32	19·2	
Sibling	244	176·1	115	107·8		115	99·0	
Child	201	64·5	41	38·5		41	32·2	
All	492	279·0	188	169·2	> 0·10	188	150·4	≅ 0·001

TABLE 8   Comparison of dominant and recessive modes of inheritance offspring of Dupuytren's × Dupuytren's mating (Thieme)

Total seen	Dominant hypothesis			Recessive hypothesis		
	Observed	Expected	P	Observed	Expected	P
44	15	15·6	> 0·80	15	20·9	< 0·05

to be better with a dominant than a recessive hypothesis. It is probably not a polygenic pattern for in these one expects the families to have a lesser number of affected relatives as seen for instance in club foot. This is not the situation in Dupuytren's.

Further evidence for the inheritance of Dupuytren's being autosomal dominant is offered by Thieme's observations in the 44 children in whom both parents had Dupuytren's (Table 8). Dominance would be expected to show 75 per cent incidence in the children; recessive inheritance with clinical expression must be homozygous and would occur in 100 per cent. The observed figures in children confirm a dominant autosomal mode of inheritance for Dupuytren's.

The population incidence of epilepsy is probably 0·5 per cent (Fairfield, 1954). In this series of 371 patients with Dupuytren's, 32, 8·4 per cent, had both diseases compared to the expected 1·86 individuals. In the epileptics, 32 patients (29 per cent) were found to have Dupuytren's. This is more than the expected incidence even though they were young individuals; 15·1 per cent would have been the expected number in this age group. Thieme was unable, however, to find evidence of undue epilepsy in the relatives of Dupuytren's patients, nor excessive Dupuytren's amongst the families of epileptics (Table 9). To date, therefore, although his figures do in fact confirm the frequency of the two diseases in combination there is as yet no proof of linked inheritance.

His final observation is that barbiturate usage is unrelated to the occurrence of Dupuytren's in epileptics as suggested by Skoog (1948).

TABLE 9   Frequencies of epilepsy in Dupuytren's index families, and of Dupuytren's in epilepsy index families (Thieme)

	Seen	Number Corrected for age	Epilepsy Found	Expected	P
First degree relatives of Dupuytren's index	492	—	8	2·46	> 0·05
			Dupuytren's Found	Expected	
First degree relatives of epilepsy index	208	100·2	18	23·3	> 0·30

	(a) Complications			(b) Complications	
	Complete fasciectomy 51 cases (per cent)	Partial fasciectomy 125 cases (per cent)	Local excision 31 cases (per cent)	Complete fasciectomy 63 cases (per cent)	Partial fasciectomy 65 cases (per cent)
Haematoma	7 7·7	4 3·1	1 3·2	2 3·2	3 4·5
Delayed wound healing	11 12·1	8 6·2	—	3 4·8	3 4·35
Persisting œdema	5 5·5	6 4·65	1 3·2	1 1·6	2 3·0
Joint reaction	3 3·2	2 1·55	1 3·2	1 1·6	1 4·5
Infection	—	1 0·77	—	—	1 4·5

Acknowledgements. I am grateful to Mr R. S. M. Ling for permission to reproduce Tables 1–4 and Figures 1–3 from his article in the *Journal of Bone and Joint Surgery,* British volume, 1963. I am grateful to the Journal also for permission.

I am grateful to Dr W. Thieme of Seattle, Washington, U.S.A., for permission to reproduce Tables 5–9.

REFERENCES

BURCH, P. R. J. (1966). Dupuytren's contracture: an auto-immune disease? *Journal of Bone and Joint Surgery*, **48-B,** 312.

EARLY, P. F. (1962). Population studies in Dupuytren's contracture. *Journal of Bone and Joint Surgery*, **41-B,** 602.

FAIRFIELD, L. (1954). *Epilepsy—Grand Mal, Petit Mal, Convulsions,* p. 30. London: Gerard Duckworth.

HUESTON, J. T. (1960). The Incidence of Dupuytren's contracture: *Medical Journal of Australia*, ii, 999.

LING, R. S. M. (1963). The genetic factor in Dupuytren's disease. *Journal of Bone and Joint Surgery*, **45-B,** 709.

LUND, M. (1941). Dupuytren's Contracture and Epilepsy. *Acta Psychiatrica et Neurologica*, **16,** 465.

SKOOG, T. (1948). Dupuytren's contraction, with special reference to aetiology and improved surgical treatment. Its occurrence in epileptics. Note on knuckle pads. *Acta Chirurgica Scandinavica*, **96,** Supplementum 139.

THIEME, W. Personal communication, 1969.

6. THE RELATIONSHIP OF TRAUMA TO DUPUYTREN'S CONTRACTURE

G. Fisk

The relationship of injury to the onset, progress or pattern of Dupuytren's contracture has been under discussion since Dupuytren, in 1832, attributed the cause of contracture in the hand of his own coachman to the pressure of the butt of his whip. Since then opinions have varied from those of Bunnell and others that injury did not cause or hasten the progress of the contracture, to those who suggested that repeated trauma, particularly to the ulnar aspect of the palm, had a significant effect. Many writers have been impressed by the progress of the disease after one episode, and Clarkson (1961) has concluded 'that a single trauma, severe or otherwise, can cause the onset of the disease in a predisposed person'. Early (1962) examining the hands of some five thousand employees at a locomotive works showed that occupation had no influence upon the onset of the disease. There appears to be strong evidence that Dupuytren's contracture is genetically determined, and we are left therefore with the question as to whether extrinsic factors play any part in the age of onset, in the pattern, distribution and progress of the deformity. It has certainly been conceded that sufferers from epilepsy, chronic alcoholism and pulmonary tuberculosis show an increased incidence and an earlier onset of the disease. It is possible that there is an associated genetic factor predisposing subjects to these conditions as well as Dupuytren's contracture, but it seems more likely that these are extrinsic factors. It must be emphasized that no variety of disease or injury, activity or occupation could induce Dupuytren's contracture in somebody who was not genetically so determined.

It seems essential to rationalize our attitude towards the influence of trauma in Dupuytren's contracture. Quite apart from its academic and therapeutic interest, the medico-legal aspect becomes important in those societies where industrial compensation can be awarded either by the State or in the Law Courts in cases of industrial injury. (Indeed under English Common Law recompense can be sought from any third party for any injury whatsoever in a civil action. As I understand it the employment of a person with a predisposition to any condition does not absolve the employer of the responsibility for the effects of the condition if these are brought on during the course of that individual's employment.) If it is conceded that trauma is an aggravating or precipitating factor, the way is open to perhaps as many as 25 per cent of the working population to make such claims, particularly if the retirement age is increased to 70 years with the slower ageing of the general population. Such a situation has already been described among New York brewery workers (Moorhead, 1953). As exponents in the field of hand surgery we are constantly asked to give our views upon this point by both workmen and employers, and it is essential to give an unbiased view based upon the available evidence.

What are the arguments against Dupuytren's contracture being caused by direct trauma to the hand? They are:

1. The condition is not seen any more commonly in manual workers than clerical workers; indeed, it is said to be slightly commoner in non-manual workers.
2. It appears bilaterally in some 40 per cent of patients and the dominant hand is not more frequently affected than the other.
3. It has a familial incidence and has been reported in identical twins.
4. It is associated with fibrous overgrowth elsewhere, knuckle pads, Peyronie's disease, plantar fascial thickening.
5. Injuries to the palmar fascia are not all followed by Dupuytren's contracture, and scarring of the palm, as for instance after burns, never follows the pattern of change and deformity seen in Dupuytren's contracture.
6. Hueston (1963) draws attention to the fact that invalids with enforced inactivity of the hands will give a history of the contracture occurring or increasing during their period of immobility.

What are the arguments in favour of trauma being an important factor?

1. It is commoner in men than women.
2. Its incidence increases steadily with age, which may indicate that chronic minor trauma to the hand has a cumulative effect.
3. It appears to be associated with injury to the hand and arm and its complications, namely after Sudeck's dystrophy (Plewes, 1956), tennis elbow (Rang, 1962), and frozen shoulder (Early, 1962).

Hueston in a personal series of 220 patients, had eleven patients who gave a convincing history of the contracture appearing soon after local injury to the hand and after injury to the arm in six further patients. He does, however, suggest that the enforced immobilization of the limb and swelling of the hand at the time may have been significant. Like many other conditions patients claim that a specific circumstance or injury brought about some disease process whereas, in fact, it merely drew the attention of the patient to the disease, and this is undoubtedly often true in Dupuytren's contracture. Many other patients in the hope of financial gain endeavour to obtain recompense on these grounds. It is significant that in a review of 122 patients with Dupuytren's disease in the Royal Air Force (Morley, 1959) twenty-five claimed a definite history of injury to the palm with almost immediate onset of contraction. It cannot escape our notice that if such claims were acceded to these airmen would be pensionable.

A recent review of the histories of sixty-six males affected by the disease, engaged predominantly in the maritime trades, showed that a total of 104 hands were involved—fifty-five right and forty-nine left. Despite the predominance of heavy manual work in this industry twenty-eight (42 per cent) of the patients could be classified as non-manual workers including a surprising number of merchant navy officers. Four subjects attributed their condition to their occupation. In twenty-two cases there was a history of previous single injury to one hand, but in thirteen of these cases the condition was bilateral. The condition was more advanced in ten cases in the injured hand, but in three the contralateral hand was worse. There were four cases claiming that a single injury had produced new or increasing contracture of the hand within a few days or weeks of the injury, but in one case the contralateral hand had more advanced deformity, and in another there was a known 3 years history. In the other eighteen cases, where there was a history of remote injury to the hand, only one case appeared to have contracture arising at the site of the scar of the laceration sustained 2 years previously.

It would seem, therefore, in this small series of 104 hands affected in sixty-six male subjects in an industry notorious for its tendency to litigate there is little or no evidence that Dupuytren's contracture has been caused or its pattern determined by previous injury. Although not statistically significant, the age of onset of the disease in these twenty-two cases did not differ from that for the whole group.

Nevertheless, it is common experience that cases are occasionally seen where the relationship between a specific injury and the onset of the contracture is quite striking. Must we therefore concede that in certain circumstances this relationship can be accepted, or is it not possible that injury to the hand and the incidence of Dupuytren's contracture, especially in the older age groups, is sufficiently common for the relationship to be coincidental?

SUMMARY

Dupuytren's contracture is an hereditary disease manifesting itself late in life, but whose course and pattern may be modified by extrinsic factors of epilepsy, pulmonary tuberculosis, chronic alcoholism and immobilization of the hand for various reasons; occupation and recurrent trauma (except as a result of the normal ageing process) has no effect upon the disease; a single injury to the hand may cause a reaction difficult to distinguish from Dupuytren's contracture or perhaps draw the patient's attention to a previously unobserved lesion, but does not itself induce Dupuytren's contracture.

REFERENCES

CLARKSON, P. (1961). *Guy's Hospital Reports*, **110**, 52.
DUPUYTREN, G. (1832). *Leçons orales de Clinique chirurgicale*, vol. 1. Paris: Baillière.
EARLY, P. F. (1962a). *Journal of Bone and Joint Surgery*, **44-B**, 602.
EARLY, P. F. (1962b). *Lancet*, 427.
HUESTON, J. T. (1962). *Medical Journal of Australia*, 1, 586.
HUESTON, J. T. (1963). *Dupuytren's Contracture*. Edinburgh: Livingstone.
MOORHEAD, J. J. (1953). *American Journal of Surgery*, **85**, 352.
MORLEY, G. (1959). Cited by Collins British Hand Clubs. Royal College of Surgeons of England, November 1959.
PLEWES, L. (1956). *Journal of Bone and Joint Surgery*, **38-B**, 195.
RANG, M. (1962). *Lancet*, i, **1**, 217.

7. EVALUATION OF DEFORMITY IN DUPUYTREN'S CONTRACTURE

R. Tubiana, J. Michon and Jean-Michel Thomine

An objective method of evaluating the lesions in Dupuytren's contracture appears necessary before measurement and comparison of surgical results can be attempted. It may also allow some degree of pre-operative assessment of prognosis.

The formula that we use takes into account not only the degree of individual digital flexion but also the distribution of lesions throughout the hand. It has been progressively revised and in particular includes suggestions by J. T. Hueston and H. Millesi.

The hand is divided into five segments, each consisting of a finger and its corresponding palmar zone, which includes the pretendinous band of the palmar aponeurosis to the four medial fingers, its adjacent segment of the main palmar aponeurosis, and its corresponding natatory ligament. The fascia of the thenar eminence and of the first web space are part of the thumb segment.

For each of these five segments the digital and palmar aponeurotic lesions are allocated a sign corresponding to a certain stage of the disease. Each stage thus represented, corresponds to the sum total of the deformity of each finger. These total deformities are measured by adding together the individual flexion deformities (deficiencies of extension) of the three joints—M.P., P.I.P. and D.I.P. When there is hyperextension of the D.I.P. the degree of hyperextension is added to the total flexion deformity of the other joints. For the thumb the loss of abduction of the first metacarpal (by comparison with the opposite thumb if it is not involved), is added to the deformities of the M.P. and I.P. joints.

Theoretically for each finger the range of deformity is from $0°$ (complete extension) to $200°$ (fixation of the finger into the palm), and from $0°$ to $160°$ for the thumb.

Thus we distinguish five stages:

Stage 0 = no lesion;

    N = palmar nodule with established flexion deformity;

    1 = total flexion deformity between $0°$ and $45°$;

    2 = total flexion deformity between $45°$ and $90°$;

    3 = total flexion deformity between $90°$ and $155°$;

    4 = total flexion deformity exceeding $135°$.

In addition a letter is added to prefix the number thus calculated for each finger.

P, for palmar, indicates that the lesions are predominantly in the palm.

D, for digital, indicates that the lesions are predominantly in the fingers. Because the flexion deformity at the P.I.P. joint is more difficult to correct than at the M.P. joint, any deformity exceeding 90 degrees at the I.P. joints is registered as D +. If the lesions are both palmar and digital, the code number is followed by P.D.

H, for hyperextension, indicates the advanced deformity with D.I.P. in fixed hyperextension.

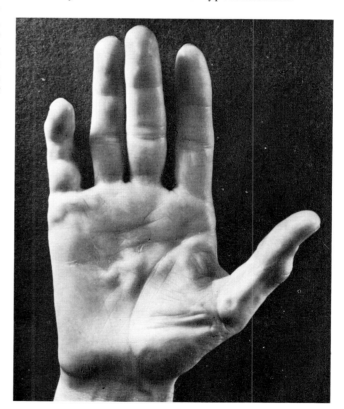

Figure 7.1
IPD = Palmar nodule without deformity; with retraction of the first web space to $45°$.
NP = Palmar nodule without retraction.
IPD = Retraction of the little finger to less than $45°$; also with nodule at the base of the little finger.
Formula: IDP, NP, NP, NP, IPD = 3·5
Total 3·5 = addition of the retractions of both thumb and little finger = 1 + 1 = 2. Then add 3 palmar nodules without retraction at the base of the central 3 fingers = 0·5 × 3 = 1·5 = total 3·5.

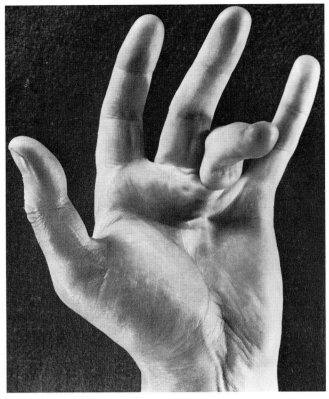

Figure 7.2
No lesion in the thumb, index, middle or little fingers. The ring finger shows 30° flexion at the metacarpophalangeal and 70° at the proximal interphalangeal level and these retractions added = 30 + 70 = 100 — stage 3. Formula O, O, O, 3PD, O.

For the specialist in hand surgery some other letters are added to lend precision to the postoperative notes.

A, for amputation.

A.A., for articular arthrodesis.

F, for fixed, indicating permanent joint stiffness and loss of flexion.

R, for true recurrence, namely the reappearance of lesions within the area already cleared at operation.

E, for extension, namely the appearance of new lesions outside the area cleared at operation.

All these representative code signs are then assembled —beginning conventionally with the thumb.

Each of the five rays of the hand is represented in turn by a number (or N) indicating the stage, followed by the appropriate relevant letters.

The rays without aponeurotic lesions are represented by o.

A concise but precise clinical assessment is thus obtained for each case.

Since the five parts of this assessment express the extent of the disease in the hand and each of the numerals expresses the degree of deformity or stage in each finger, it is now possible to represent the total state of the disease process in the hand by adding together the numerals of each of the individual formulae. Rather than ignore an aponeurotic lesion without deformity, stage N is allocated 0·5.

A hand with Dupuytren's contracture can thus be represented by a specific formula, theoretically extending from 0·5 (nodule without deformity) to 20 (all five fingers flexed to stage 4).

The assessment formula is worked out before

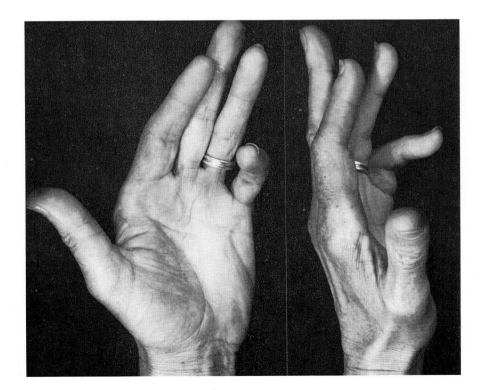

Figure 7.3
No lesion on the thumb or the middle finger; a nodule in the proximal phalanx of the index producing proximal interphalangeal flexion less than 45°; a palmar nodule at the base of the ring finger without any deformity; and a proximal interphalangeal deformity of the little finger of 90° (D+) with hyperextension of the terminal phalanx (H). Formula O, ID, O, NP, 3D+, H.

wavy course followed by the fibre bundles. Under longitudinal tension the waviness is smoothed out and transverse striation disappears. When tension is released the previous state is resumed. In 14 palmar aponeuroses some of the fibre bundles even in the relaxed state had lost their waviness and transverse striation, but the fibre bundles were still slender and well demarcated. In 20 specimens, whereas individual fibre bundles presented similar changes, the bundles were, in addition, thickened. Twelve specimens showed, together with the changes just described, a tendency on the part of the thickened fibre bundles to fuse together in individual places, and to form larger bundles. So much for the changes as seen under illumination with the loupe. Histological sections showed increased collagen in the changed fibre bundles compared with the normal (Fig. 8.1). The elastic fibres were no longer

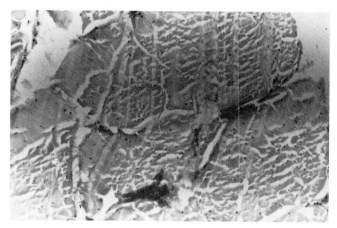

Figure 8.2
Haematoxilin-eosin (1:100). Thickened collagen fibres in cross section. The single collagen fibres are thickened and show tendency to fusion.

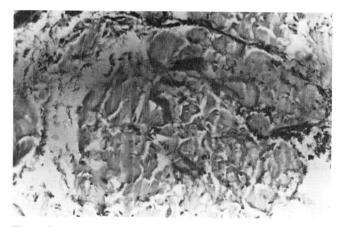

Figure 8.1
Elastica after Pranter (1:100).

evenly distributed in the fibre bundle but were situated only sparcely on the periphery. The individual collagen fibres in the bundles were thickened and tended to fuse together. The thick bundles structure, especially the perifascicular connective tissue separating the bundles from one another, were normal (Fig. 8.2). In the 12 specimens, where, under the magnifier, fusion of bundles had been observed in individual places, in the histological sections numerous areas which could be interpreted as cell proliferation were observed, but always only within those fibre bundles which had undergone pathological change. The changes described fitted in perfectly with the features in the nine specimens macroscopically identified as D.C.

The contention that the changes described have a real relationship with D.C. is supported by the following considerations:

1. Individual fibre bundles were always the only ones concerned, while the remainder of the bundle in each specimen presented a normal picture, so

that an artefact or a diffuse change within the definition of senile degeneration could be excluded.

2. The distribution of the changes in the finger rays nearly corresponds to the distribution in D.C. It was as follows:

Middle finger ray	12 times
Ring finger ray	34 times
Little finger ray	28 times

3. Only longitudinal fibres were affected; transverse fibres never affected (Fig. 8.3) (Skoog, 1966).

4. The male sex was predominant.

5. The findings form an uninterrupted line from the early changes to the fully developed picture of D.C.

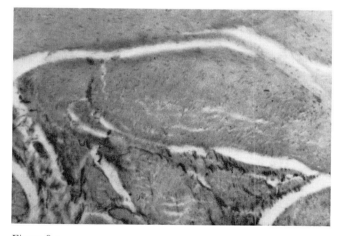

Figure 8.3
Elastica after Pranter (1:100). Longitudinal section. The thickened collagen fibre bundle does not contain elastic fibres. In the lower part the normal fibre bundles of the transverse fibre system show elastic fibres in normal number and distribution.

As soon as these early changes had been recognized, it was not difficult to discover them again and identify them in the operation specimens, in which they could be demonstrated in the places where the disease was invading healthy tissue.

With the above observations in mind we believe that D.C. commences with changes in the collagen fibres in the fibre bundles of the tense connective system on the volar aspect of the hand. With a previous history of a sufficiently significant hereditary component any fibre bundle can be the site of pathological change. The processes of ageing and functional stress are predisposing factors. The collagen fibres thicken, fuse together

Histologically the bundle structure and perifascicular connective tissue are preserved. Up to this point the changes could be described as the *stage of fibre thickening*.

Commencing from the perivascular areas, proliferation of fibroblasts develops in the fibre bundles which have undergone the pathological changes described above. The cells gradually invade the whole cross-section of the fibre bundle, and the collagen substance disappears. Under the electron microscope the microfibril bundles can be seen dissolving (Fig. 8.4). At commencement of cell proliferation the septa of perifascicular connective tissue between the fibre bundles remain intact (Fig. 8.5). During proliferation however,

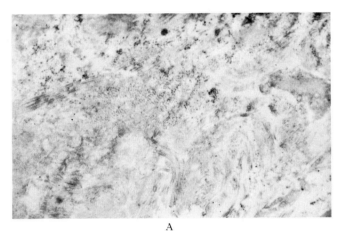

A

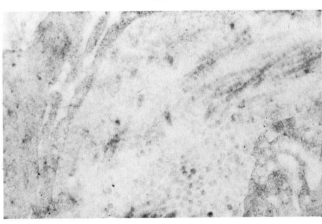

B

Figure 8.4
Fixation Glutaminosmiumsaure. Electron microscope 1 : 5000 (A); 1 : 25000 (B). Tissue of a contracture band during early cellular proliferation. The collagen microfibril bundles in dissolution.

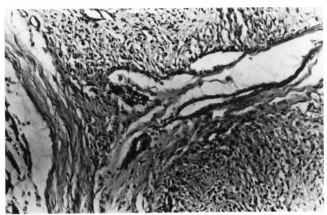

Figure 8.5
Haematoxilin-Eosin (1 : 100). Two pathologic fibre bundles in cross section. Early cellular proliferation. The perifascicular connective tissue and the septa between the bundles still intact.

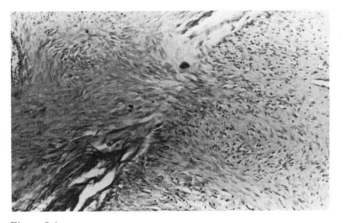

Figure 8.6
Elastica after Pranter (1:100). Two pathologic fibre bundles in cross section during cellular proliferation. The fibre bundles still separated by a septum. The septum is being destroyed by the cellular proliferation.

and as a result there is a thickening of the whole fibre bundle as the next higher structure. The bundle loses the property of assuming the wavy state when it is relaxed. On account of this thickening the space between the fibre bundles decreases, and with the aid of the loupe only they become frequently difficult to delineate.

the septa are perforated (Fig. 8.6) and disintegrate. If parts of the perifascicular connective tissue become enclosed between two fibre bundles in the process of fusing together, the pictures are confused.

Intact connective tissue together with intact elastic fibres can be situated in the middle of a contracture band. The real state of affairs can only be cleared up by examination of a series of sections. At the peak of cell proliferation, the bundle structure has disappeared. A thicker band has developed which in cross-section is mainly occupied by fibroblasts. Longitudinal and serial examination can still reveal the origin of the band through the fusion of a number of fibre bundles.

During further development of the process the cells mature with the formation of precollagen and collagen. The cell count decreases and the mass of intermediate substance increases. The collagen substance is not, from a functional point of view, constructed in regular fibres and fibre bundles, but appears as strata, in a vertiforme arrangement or, in a form resembling a spindle. This period can be regarded as the stage of *cell-maturation and fibre production.*

The development just described results in a scar-like picture. There are now only a few more mature fibrocytes to be seen. The tissue consists of collagen substance in either stratified or spindleform arrangements. We are concerned here with the stage which conforms with the fibrous or lamella stage in the classical descriptions. If only a few sections are available for histological examination, the picture can be confused with the stage of fibre-thickening, because the appearances are similar. Differentiation depends on an evaluation of the perifascicular connective tissue. If this is present, the process is in the stage of fibre-thickening. If the perifascicular connective tissue, together with the bundle structure, has disappeared, we are then concerned with the *fibrous stage.*

In fibre bundles which have passed through all the developmental stages and have reached the stage of scar tissue, cell proliferation can recommence. The whole process—cell proliferation, distintegration of collagen, cell maturation, renewed collagen production can possibly be repeated many times. The possibility of this repetitive process is the cause of the stop–go course of the disease, alternating between periods of activity and inactivity. The clinical course on that account also becomes irregular, because in different places in the tense connective tissue system on the volar aspect of the hand, different stages of the disease process can be present at the same time. The identification of these secondary and tertiary stages is naturally difficult, and can only succeed with absolute certainty if sections in two planes are available, so that a special picture of the arrangement of the tissue can be constructed.

Round cell infiltration which is regarded in the literature as an expression of an inflammatory component of the disease, was not regularly seen. According to Nezelof and Tubiana (1958), and also Larsen and Posch (1958) this occurs in only about 25 per cent of cases, a frequency too small to be of pathogenetic significance. They occur in large numbers where fatty tissue or sweat glands become involved between thickening fibre bundles, and undergo pressure atrophy. We interpret the round cell infiltration as being a re-absorptive inflammatory reaction.

Iron pigment deposits which are occasionally met with, have been considered as being the expression of the termination of haemorrhages, and have been put forward as an argument in favour of the traumatic genesis of D.C. (Skoog, 1948). They can, however, occur within the framework of the tissue transformation described above, and should not be overrated as conclusive evidence.

Operation specimens from 176 cases were examined, with regard to their stage in the disease, by means of sections in two planes and in some cases by series of sections. The determination of the average duration of the pathological changes produced a striking conformity between the histological picture and the duration of the disease. The mean periods were as follows:

Stage of fibre thickening	4 years
Stage of cell proliferation	5·66 years
Stage of fibre production	6·2 years
Fibrous stage	7·55 years
Secondary cell proliferation	10·3 years

Summarizing these morphological investigations, the conclusions are as follows. D.C. is the manifestation of pathological changes in the fibres and fibre bundles of the tense collagen connective tissue system of the volar aspect of the hand. The pathological tissue arises through the transformation of existing fibres and fibre bundles and not by neoformation. Fundamentally any fibre in the system can be subject to this pathological change, and this is confirmed by clinical analysis of the distribution of pathological variations in the hand. Individual fibre systems are of course affected due to specific causes, partly not understood, and in varying frequency. Some form of systemic disease is consequently involved. A comparison between the morphological process and the time factor shows that the course of the disease extends over many years and can always recommence.

THE NATURAL COURSE OF D.C.

As already mentioned, all individual studies of the untreated course of D.C. are contrary to the concept of an unbroken continuity in the progress of the disease, but recognize on the contrary an irregular phasic course for each individual case. An understanding of the natural course of D.C. can only be achieved if a large reservoir of patients is followed up over a considerable length of time and every sign of activity recorded. The following would be regarded as signs of activity.

Appearance of a nodule or band on a site previously free of changes.

Appearance of a flexion contracture within the area of a band which previously had caused no finger contraction.

The worsening of an existing finger contracture.

It is obvious that an assessment is only possible if an exact description of the status was made on the first examination. It is equally clear that such an examination cannot determine the precise activity of the disease, because changes which are a manifestation of early activity but which are below the threshold of recognition on examination for the case record, escape evaluation. For example it is difficult to be precise about the increase in the thickness of a contracture band or nodule. Similarly the increase of an existing flexion contracture from, for example, 40° over a matter of one or two degrees is difficult to determine with the measuring technique at present in use. Hence only recordable differences will be recorded. As long as there is an adequate degree of uniformity in case assessment no harm will have been done to the result.

The percentage of cases in a patient reservoir which manifests activity in the sense described above, is termed the activity rate. Should the reservoir contain a large number of cases with marked predisposition—the expression 'Dupuytren's diathesis' is employed—and a larger activity rate must be expected than when the reverse holds good. It can, however, be accepted that with a sufficiently large number of cases there will be a smoothing out in the overall composition. Inquiry was first directed to the course of the disease in 150 hands which on examination for the first time presented either a nodule or a band on the palm of finger, without any contraction (Stage 'O'). In these cases operation was not called for and no special treatment was given. Activity rate in relation to time of observation was:

3 to 5 years   37   per cent
6 to 12 years   46·5 per cent

In nine hands during the period of observation there was temporary involution of nodules or bands originally present in the hands. Given an adequate length of observation time, no case of involution was permanent.

A follow-up of 47 cases recently carried out, in which there was no flexion contracture (Stage 'O'), and which were given conservative treatment such as X-ray, vitamin E or ultra-sonic sound, resulted in a similar activity rate (Hassler, 1967) from which the conclusion may be drawn that the course of the disease was not significantly influenced by these methods.

In a further study the fate of 113 hands was followed, in which at the first examination there were no signs of the disease. The patients were being treated for D.C. in the contralateral hand. In the course of time a proportion of the hands originally free of the disease became affected to the following extent:

With an observation time of 5 years   39 per cent
With an observation time of 6 to 12 years   48 per cent

Similar results were found in this investigation when other postulates were used.

If a large group of patients is investigated in which there is more or less advanced flexion contracture, difficulties arise, and not because an actual flexion is easier to determine than a gradually increasing flexion, but because the presence of flexion contracture is an indication for operation and the operation cannot be delayed on investigational grounds. Some criterion as to the activity of the disease can obviously be achieved indirectly, namely as follows. In a large group of patients the duration of the disease is determined as accurately as possible. The cases are arranged in several groups according to the length of the history. The percentage of cases with mild, moderate, or severe flexion in each case is noted. The percentage of moderate or severe cases increases in the course of time. A criterion as to the activity of the disease can be obtained by the rise in the moderate and severe cases. From this system of grouping a picture emerges showing that the activity rate increases in proportion to the number of severe cases in a group (Fig. 8.7).

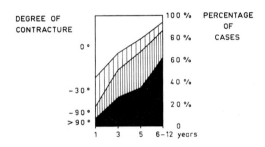

Figure 8.7
In a series of 221 cases the degree of contracture of the most involved digit is plotted against duration of the disease in years. This gives an indirect approach to the progression of the disease in advanced cases.

Investigations regarding the natural course of D.C. justify the following conclusion.

The individual case of D.C. displays a phasic course with periods of inactivity and progress. Prediction regarding the future course of the disease is not possible in an individual case. Only evaluation of a large patient reservoir can elucidate its progress. If such a reservoir is available for homogeneous patient material, the activity rate is shown to be remarkably constant. Its time relationship can be represented by a curve. Activity rate increases with the lapse of time, more rapidly during the first four or five years, but always perceptibly. The activity rate further depends on the medium grade of severity of the disease. The activity rate is higher where a greater number of severe cases are included in the clinical material.

The results of these investigations on the natural course of D.C. are of the greatest significance in the evaluation of treatment. Adequate assessment of investigations relative to treatment can only be achieved by appropriate consideration of the natural course of the disease.

EVALUATION OF RESULTS OF TREATMENT

An objective evaluation of the results of treatment must be based on two assessments entirely independent of one another.

Furthermore the information they contain must be sufficiently complete if they are to be of adequate value.

1. FUNCTIONAL CONDITION OF THE HAND

The resulting function of the hand depends on various factors not immediately associated with one another. If a severe flexion contracture has already existed for some time, there can be secondary tendon contracture or stiffening of the joints. The functional result can be prejudiced by this, although the post-operative course of events may be free of complications and recurrence. On the other hand serious postoperative complications can be the cause of a bad result, although there is no further D.C. activity. Finally an excellent postoperative result can be ruined by renewed activity of D.C. whether in the form of either a recurrence, or an extension of the complaint into a hitherto healthy area. The functional condition can be expressed most simply by the degree of flexion and extension of the finger worst affected.

2. ACTIVITY OF D.C.

Following operation further activity of the disease can make its appearance in two ways. New pathological tissue can develop within the scene of the preceding operation (recurrence), or contracture tissue can appear in an area originally healthy and with which the operation was not concerned (extension). This new development of contracture tissue can result once again in flexion contracture, and the functional state of the hand deteriorates. It is possible for a band or nodule to be present without causing a contracture and which is therefore overlooked in functional assessment. In the evaluation of results of treatment, activity of the disease must be emphasized, because it is only the rate of activity in relation to the progress to be expected which denotes a real therapeutic influence on the disease.

Finally, a contracture band, functionally insignificant at the time of examination, has the property for potential progress leading to a deterioration of function.

The functional condition of clinical material and its activity rate can be evaluated only if it is considered within the context of the factors in general in which activity and its results depend, these include:

1. The classification of clinical material in relation to its appropriate grade of contracture.

2. The lapse of time since operation or treatment.

The value of a report on the results of treatment is still further enhanced if the findings on two or more examinations carried out within some specified period of time are analysed. In this way a report can be made not only in regard to some specified date but also in regard to the pattern of development.

The anatomical picture of recurrences is significant in two respects. In the first place there is a fundamental difference in the anatomical structure of the tense connective tissue system on the volar aspect of the hand in the area of the palm, and on the volar aspect of the fingers. In the palm the fibrous system is anatomically much better defined than on the fingers where the distribution of fibres is diffuse. There is a difference also in regard to an operation which may eventually be necessary on account of recurrence. The removal of a recurrent nodule on a finger undoubtedly involves a far less extensive undertaking than the reopening of the palm. Information on the anatomical condition of recurrences and extensions is therefore desirable.

On the other hand information on the frequency and types of complications is of less significance in so far as the assessment of long-term results is concerned, because complications which cause a lasting influence on function become apparent in the evaluation of the functional state. As, however, complications not leading to permanent deterioration of function cause a prolonged postoperative disability this factor obviously plays an important part in the comparison between various methods of treatment. Records on the type and frequency of complications should therefore be made.

An attempt will now be made to put into effect the above principles in a group of 395 patients who underwent operation on their hands for D.C. The average time since the date of operation was 4·8 years. As regards operation, four different procedures were employed. As there are frequently confusing reports in the literature regarding precise operation procedures, exact definitions are necessary.

Fasciotomy signifies an open or closed transverse division of a contracture band without removal of the tissue. The immediate postoperative result is as a rule very good, but the entire pathological tissue remains *in situ*.

By *local excision* we mean the excision of the contracture band without extending the operation into neighbouring healthy tissue. The operation is limited to pathological tissue and is believed* to be identical with so-called 'limited fasciectomy' (Hueston, 1963), but we avoid the expression fasciectomy as the ending 'ectomy' in general usage denotes the removal of a structure to which this particular word ending is attached, in this case 'fasci'. In limited fasciectomy, however, the healthy remote parts of the fascia remain

*Wrongly, Ed. (J.T.H.).

where they are and it is closer to a 'partial fasciectomy'.

Fasciectomy means the removal of the palmar fascia with all its processes and indeed not only diseased but also healthy tissue. Fasciectomy can be limited to the ulnar side of the palm, in which case we are dealing with a *partial fasciectomy*. In spite of this transverse limitation, removal of the palmar fascia within the scene of operation is carried out without regard to whether the tissue is diseased or not. Finally fasciectomy can include the whole of the palm. We describe this as *complete fasciectomy*. The expression 'radical' should be avoided, as it has a special connotation in relation to the surgery of tumours, and is out of context in the field of D.C.

Fasciotomy was performed on only 9 of the 395 patients.

In all these 9 hands the postoperative result was very good, and the function of the hand notably improved. In a follow-up of 3 to 5 years eight of the nine hands had deteriorated considerably from a functional point of view, and was the same or even worse than the preoperative status. We soon abandoned this procedure, so that the number of cases has remained small.

The results of the three other procedures are shown in Fig. 8.8. On the left of each column the preoperative

(Stage 'O') and where following operation extension was only possible up to $175°$, in other words a deterioration of $5°$, must be placed in the fourth group (no improvement or deterioration) and not in the group $0°$ to $150°$. Cases should only be placed in this group if there is an improvement in function.

The figure shows that partial fasciectomy led to more unfavourable clinical results because this group comprised more advanced cases. In spite of this, however, the functional results are better than in the local excision group. The two groups complete fasciectomy and local excision comprise cases with a comparable functional state before operation. The difference in the percentage of unfavourable results is correspondingly marked. It must be emphasized that the immediate postoperative results of these two groups were equally good, and that the difference only emerged over the years during the development of recurrences and extensions. A follow-up a short time after operation would not have recorded the difference.

Figure 8.9 is a summary of the activity rate in the three groups. The left-hand side of the columns shows the rate after three to five years, and the right-hand side after six to twelve years. The development of functional

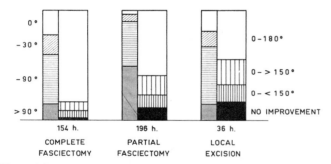

Figure 8.8
The functional results of three different methods are compared. The mean observation time is 4·8 years. It is equal in the 3 groups of patients. On the left side of each column the functional state before operation is shown.

functional conditions are set out. Four groups are differentiated according to the degree of flexion contracture of the finger worst affected. On the right-hand side the functional states are set out in relation to the follow-up, namely after an average of 4·8 years. Here also there are four different groups. Three of them include all cases with complete flexion and in which there is an improvement in relation to the preoperative condition. They are classified according to the degree of limitation of extension of the worst finger. The fourth group comprises all cases where there is flexion deficiency and cases where the functional condition at the time of follow-up was either the same as the preoperative condition or had become even worse. A hand which before operation had completely normal extension

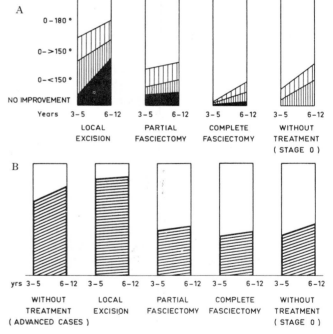

Figure 8.9
Functional state in relation to time of follow up. This figure represents the cases with a follow up of more than 3 years. The functional result after 3 to 5 years and after a follow up of 6 to 12 years is compared to show the progression of the disease from the functional point of view (A).

Rate of activity in relation of time. In Figure 9 B the percentage of cases showing any sign of activity of the disease after 3 to 5 years (left side of each column) and after 6 to 12 years (right side) is represented.

results for the same periods can be read from the shaded parts of each column.

The activity rate of the complete fasciectomy group was 35 per cent after 3 to 5 years and 39 per cent after 6 to 12 years. For the partial fasciectomy groups the corresponding figures are 40 per cent and 44 per cent respectively. If these figures are compared with the untreated cases in stage 'O', for which the corresponding figures are 37 per cent and 46 per cent, the conformity is striking. The activity rate of an untreated group similar to the complete fasciectomy group as regards severity, is found to be 66 per cent for the 3 to 5 year period and 79 per cent for the 6 to 12 year period. The activity rate for an untreated group corresponding to partial fasciectomy grouping must be even higher still. By making use of these two procedures in operation not only was the functional condition of the hands in regard to their eventual condition markedly improved, but the progress of the disease was altered in such a way that the group concerned reverted to stage 'O' and the disease was, so to speak, brought back to the original point from which it started. It is most certainly not to be expected that the disease can be completely extinguished by operation, as we are concerned with a systemic disease and even after very extensive operations sufficient connective tissue is left behind and can become subject to the same pathological change. Reports of successes which reveal either an insignificant or zero percentage of cases with active disease are completely unreliable. The difference in the two groups of complete and partial fasciectomies as regards activity rate is small. It is immediately evident, however, if the anatomical situation regarding persistent D.C. activity is brought into account. The majority of recurrences and extensions following complete fasciectomy occurred in the fingers, only 7·7 per cent being in the palm. Following partial fasciectomy on the other hand, the palm was concerned in 78·6 per cent of the recurrences and extensions. The more extensive operation (complete fasciectomy) could not, admittedly, reduce activity in the finger regions in relation to the less extensive operation, but does, however, to a large extent prevent recurrence in the palm.

As regards local excision, Figure 8 shows the marked increase in unfavourable results after more than 5 years of observation. But at 86 per cent the activity rate even after 3 to 5 years is very high, though the rise after that is less significant. The activity rate is higher than an assessment for a comparative group of untreated cases in a corresponding analysis structure might be expected, namely 66–79 per cent. It should of course not be forgotten that the number of cases in this group is small, and that the figures read from them are not absolute. Perhaps there would be a smoothing out of the percentage content with an assessment of a larger group. When, however, it became clear, without reference to statistical considerations, that the results in this group would be worse, we immediately discontinued this operative procedure. Although it can be stated that following local excision the condition of the hands was materially improved it was not possible to influence the progress of D.C. On account of the activity which remains, the average improvement declines from year to year. The palm was involved in all recurrences and extensions in this group.

The percentage figures for complications can be seen in Table I. The frequency of complications is more or less equally distributed over the three groups. A higher incidence was only recorded in regard to haematomata in the complete fasciectomy group, which it was possible to reduce by means of improvement in incisions, a stricter approach to the indications for operation, and by suction drainage.

DISCUSSION

From an evaluation of the results of the above investigation, the following points emerge for discussion:
1. The study of early development of D.C. shows that in the first place there is a pathological change in

TABLE I Percentage of complications

	A					B		
	Complete Fasciectomy 51 cases		Partial Fasciectomy 125 cases		Local Excision 31 cases		Complete Fasciectomy 63 cases		Partial Fasciectomy 65 cases
Haematoma	7	7·7 per cent	4	3·1 per cent	I	3·2 per cent	2	3·2 per cent	3	4·5 per cent
Delayed wound healing	II	12·1 per cent	8	6·2 per cent	—		3	4·8 per cent	3	4·35 per cent
Persisting œdema	5	5·5 per cent	6	4·65 per cent	I	3·2 per cent	I	1·6 per cent	2	3·0 per cent
Joint reaction	3	3·2 per cent	2	1·55 per cent	I	3·2 per cent	I	1·6 per cent	I	1·5 per cent
Infection	—		I	0·77 per cent	—		—		I	1·5 per cent

The total number for each complication is counted. As several patients were involved with several complications the total number of complications is higher than the number of patients involved.

A presents the percentage of complications without using suction drainage.

B presents two series of cases operated upon by improved technique; Suction drainage was regularly used and a new skin incision adopted. In advanced cases the complete fasciectomy was not carried out.

the fibre bundles of the tense connective tissue system on the volar aspect of the hand. Cell proliferation then takes place within these fibres already affected. This cell proliferation has been hitherto regarded as the starting point of D.C. The tense connective tissue system of the volar aspect of the hand includes not only the palmar aponeurosis in the strict sense of the term, but all the tense connective tissue rays which are to be found on the volar aspect of the fingers and in the palm. The anatomical arrangement of the individual parts of this system have been the subject of frequent and detailed study, latterly by Stack (1967). A comparative study of the arrangement of the contracture bands among a very large group of patients with D.C. and the arrangement of the fibre bundles of the tense connective tissue system in anatomical specimens present a striking conformity (Millesi, 1959; Stack, 1967). The individual parts of the tense connective tissue system of the volar aspect of the hand are affected in D.C. in varying rates of incidence, in which functional stress would appear to be a predisposing factor. Fundamentally, however, any part may be involved. In patients with a strong tendency to progressive D.C. a large part of the connective tissue system is invaded by the disease in the course of time. From these considerations one must conclude that a prophylactic removal of parts of the tense connective tissue system not yet affected, wherever this is anatomically feasible, in other words over the whole area of the aponeurosis is rational and that this procedure reduces the possibility of further extension of the disease.

2. An analysis of the process of morphological changes reveals the possibility of a phasic development of the disease, as is also clearly recognizable in the clinical field. Following the pathological process in the collagen fibres (fibre thickening during which the actual bundle structure is preserved), cell proliferation commences. The cells mature and produce collagen fibres, no longer arranged from a functional standpoint. The bundle structure is lost, resulting in fibrous tissue with a poor cell count and in which a renewed secondary cell proliferation can develop. The whole process repeats itself. Multiple repetitions appear to be conceivable. A conception such as this in relation to the morphological development provides conformity between the histological picture and the clinical course of the disease. It provides a closely woven background for the clinical observation that D.C. can become active again after many years of inactivity.

3. The comparision between the average clinical and histological pictures leads to the concept of continuing and repeated stages building up into a disease of very many years duration. Cases which manifest histologically a picture of secondary cell proliferation, have a previous history of the disease of more than ten years. Repeated activity of D.C. can accordingly occur

after many years. The assumption that the disease in any way comes to an end cannot be justified by any morphological argument. A worthwhile assessment of the disease by means of a single follow-up examination after a relatively short time is therefore not possible. Only a long-term follow-up programme associated with a large mass of clinical material permits conclusion regarding the average progress of the disease, thereby providing a picture with some semblance of reality.

4. The inventory of successes recorded by various authors following treatment of D.C. by various methods discloses markedly contradictory reports. While the sincerity of individual observations is not to be doubted, there must be something wrong with the organization of the system of assessment. If well balanced regard is not paid to the important factors having a marked bearing on the results of a followup programme comparable and objective findings cannot be expected. The time which has elapsed since treatment is one such factor. If D.C., as morphological research has demonstrated, can become active again after ten or more years, only an observation time extending over very many years can give a really clear picture. For purposes of comparison an equally long period of time is called for. The opinion that the majority of recurrences and extensions occur within two years after operation (Hueston, 1963) cannot be confirmed. In our clinical material 48 per cent of recurrences and 44·7 per cent of extensions occurred later than three years after operation. A follow-up after three years would thus have spotted only about half of the cases.

5. A group of 150 hands in Stage 'O' (band or nodule without flexion contracture) was observed, untreated, for some considerable length of time, in order to get an insight into the natural course of the disease. After an observation period of 3 to 5 years 37 per cent of the cases manifested activity of the disease, and 46·5 per cent after 6 to 12 years. For more advanced stages progress was determined on the basis of information on cases with histories of equal duration and in respect of their functional condition. The percentage number of cases manifesting activity (the activity rate) is higher the more advanced the cases are in the clinical material under investigations. The distribution over the various stages of D.C. should be detailed in a follow-up investigation because it is only by this means that the functional results can be properly evaluated.

6. An evaluation of our own clinical material was carried out with the above factors in mind. The immediate postoperative result was predominantly influenced by the severity of the contracture and by the length of time since contracture had commenced, that is to say by the secondary changes in tendons and joints. Complications were distributed evenly over the various procedures of operation. A high rate of haematomata which at first occurred in the complete fasciectomies

was reduced by improvements in technique. The average long-term result was not materially influenced by complications. The functional result gradually deteriorated, over the course of a period of observation of many years, by the appearance of recurrences and extensions. The number of cases manifesting deterioration rose only slowly following partial and complete fasciectomy, but steeply following local excision. The activity rate following complete and partial fasciectomy corresponded approximately to the activity rate of cases in stage 'O', although, preoperatively speaking, the greater part of the clinical material consisted of more advanced cases. On the other hand activity rate following local excision was the same as was to be expected in the preoperative arrangement of the clinical group. Although there was a similar activity rate following partial and complete fasciectomy, it was noticeable that following complete fasciectomy recurrences and extensions occurred almost only in the fingers, whereas following partial fasciectomy the palm was very frequently involved. From these findings one is forced to conclude that long-term results are very much influenced by the method and extent of operation, and that prophylactic removal of originally healthy parts of the palmar aponeurosis contributes to an improvement in the long-term result by reducing the amount of tissue which is potentially liable to pathological changes.

The majority of reports of successes in the literature following treatment of D.C. reveal too short a period of observation. A recent report has appeared, however, on 73 hands (Hakstian, 1966) which had been operated on by Sir Archibald McIndoe using the method introduced by him, namely radical fasciectomy. The period of observation was 11·1 years. The gradual deterioration of the average functional condition, due to the appearance of recurrences and extensions, emerges from the tables prepared by Hakstian. In this clinical material the activity rate amounted to 51 per cent, thus

being not significantly above 46·5 per cent which we were able to establish for a group of cases in stage 'O'. Our group was evaluated between 6 and 12 years after the first examination. The average period of observation is thus lower than Hakstian's. With an exactly similar period of observation our figures would probably be the same as his. The conformity is, however, obvious without reference to the difference in time of observation. The cases which underwent fasciectomy by McIndoe show a progression similar to our fasciectomy cases as characteristic for stage 'O', although, preoperatively, they were for the most part in the more advanced stages. Discussion on the relative merits of fasciectomy and local excision will only have scientific backing when the advocates of local excision can report on this method over eleven years of equally good long-term results.

The fact that Hakstian in his follow-up arrived at the same percentage figures in activity rates is regarded by us as confirmation of our own investigations into the natural course of the disease.

SUMMARY

Investigations into the morphology of early pathological changes in Dupuytren's contracture leads to the author's own presentation. This demonstrates better than previous theories the conformity with the clinical course. The natural course of Dupuytren's contracture is investigated by observations on untreated cases. The conclusions are evaluated for the purpose of improving the system of assessment of postoperative results.

Acknowledgement. I am very grateful to my colleague M. Stephen Musgrave, who has done the translation of my paper into English, for his excellent work.

REFERENCES

ADAMS, W. (1878). Contraction of the fingers (Dupuytren's contracture) and its successful treatment by subcutaneous divisions of the palmar fascia and immediate extension. *British Medical Journal*, i, 928.

ASTITZ, J. M. A. & VINAN, O. A. A. (1959). Technik der Aponeurosectomie bei der D.K. *Prensa médica argentina*, **46**, 518.

BASSOT, J. (1969). Treatment of Dupuytren's disease by the means of pharmacodynamic ablation: physiobiological, technical bases. *Gazette des Hôpitaux de Paris*, 1969.

BUFF, H. U. (1958). Indikationen, Gefahren und Technik der operativen Behandlung der D.K. *Therapeutische Umsschau und medizinische Bibliographie*, **15**, 238.

CLARKSON, P. (1962). The radical fasciectomy operation for Dupuytren's contracture. A condemnation. Meeting of the Second Hand Club, Paris, May 1962.

CONWAY, H. (1954). Dupuytren's contracture. *American Journal of Surgery*, **87**, 101.

CONWAY, H. & STARK, R. B. (1955). Die artielle Versorgung der Weichteile der Hand. *Journal of Bone and Joint Surgery*, **36A**, 670.

DAESCHLER, E. (1903). Uber die Dupuytren'sche Palmarfascienkontraktur. Inaugural Dissertation, Munich.

DAVIS, A. A. (1932). The treatment of Dupuytren's contracture. A review of 31 cases, with an assessment of the comparative value of different methods of treatment. *British Journal of Surgery*, **19**, 539.

DICKIE, W. R. & HUGHES, N. C. (1967). Dupuytren's contracture. A review of the late results of radical fasciectomy. *British Journal of Plastic Surgery*, **20**, 311–314.

GOSSET, J. (1966). Anatomie des aponévroses palmo-digitales. *Maladie de Dupuytren*. Paris: Expansion Scientifique Française.

GOSSET, J. (1951). Le traitment de la maladie de Dupuytren avec la technique de McIndoe. *Memoires de l'Academie de Chirurgie*, **77**, 312.

GOSSET, J. & LEROUX, M. (1958). Sur le traitement de la maladie de Dupuytren. *Memoires de l'Academie de Chirurgie*, **84**, 1004.

GOSSET, J. & LEROUX, M. (1959). Sur le traitement de la maladie de Dupuytren. *Annales de Chirurgie*, **13**, 989.

GORDON, S. D. (1957). Dupuytren's contracture: recurrences and extension following surgical treatment. *British Journal of Plastic Surgery*, **9**, 286–288.

GORDON, S. D. (1963). Dupuytren's contracture. The use of free skin grafts in treatment, pp. 963–967 in *Transactions of the 3rd Congress of Plastic Surgery*. Amsterdam: Excerpta Medica Foundation.

GONZALES, R. J. Page 630 in *Transactions of the 5th Congress of the International Confederation for Plastic and Reconstructive Surgery*.

HAKSTIAN, R. W. (1966). Long term results of extensive fasciectomy. *British Journal of Plastic Surgery*, **19**, 140.

HAMLIN, E. (1951). Limited excision of D.C. *Annals of Surgery*, **134**, 94.

HAMLIN, E. (1952). Limited fasciectomy for D.C. *Annals of Surgery*, **135**, 94.

HASSLER, G. Personal communication.

HEINEMANN, G. & LUZIUS, H. (1961). Zur operativen Behandlung der Dupuytren'schen Kontraktur. *Chirurgie*, **32**, 244.

HUESTON, J. T. (1961). Limited fasciectomy for Dupuytren's contracture. *Plastic and Reconstructive Surgery*, **27**, 569–585.

HUESTON, J. T. (1962). Digital Wolfe grafts in recurrent Dupuytren's contracture. *Plastic and Reconstructive Surgery*, **29**, 342–344.

HUESTON, J. T. (1963). *Dupuytren's Contracture*. Edinburgh: Livingstone.

HUESTON, J. T. (1965). Dupuytren's contracture: the trend to conservatism. *Annals of the Royal College of Surgeons of England*, **36**, 134–151.

HUESTON, J. T. (1969). The control of recurrent Dupuytren's contracture by skin replacement. *British Journal of Plastic Surgery*, **22**, 152–156.

HUFFSTADT, A. J. C. (1952). Chirurgische Behandlung van de Contractur van Dupuytren. *Nederlands tijdschrift voor geneeskunde*, **96**, 2483.

ISELIN, M. & DICKMANN, G. D. (1951). Traitment de la maladie de Dupuytren par plastie totale en Z. *Presse médicale*, **59**, 1394.

JAMES, J. & TUBIANA, R. (1952). La maladie de Dupuytren. *Revue de Chirurgie orthopédique et réparatrice de l'Appareil moteur*, **38**, 352.

KRAFT, D. & MILLESI, H. Personal communication.

LANGSTONE, G. R. & COWAN, R. J. (1955). Dupuytren's contracture. *Journal of the International College of Surgeons*, **23**, 710.

LARSEN, R. D. & POSCH, J. L. (1958). Dupuytren's contracture. *Journal of Bone and Joint Surgery*, **40A**, 773.

LE CHUITON, M. (1957). Traitement de la maladie de Dupuytren par tendo-aponeurotomie du long palmaire. *Mémoires de l'Academie de Chirurgie*, **83**, 930.

LUCK, J. V. (1959). Dupuytren's contracture. *Journal of Bone and Joint Surgery*, **41A**, 635.

LEXER, E. (1931). Die gesamte Wiederherstellungschirurgie, 2nd edn., vol. 2, p. 837.

MASON, L. M. (1952). Dupuytren's contracture. *Archives of Surgery*, **65**, 457.

McINDOE, A. & BEARE, R. L. (1958). The surgical treatment of Dupuytren's contracture. *American Journal of Surgery*, **95**, 197.

MEYERDING, H. W. (1936). Dupuytren's contracture. *Archives of Surgery*, **32**, 320.

MILLESI, H. (1959). Neue Gesichtspunkte in der Pathogenese der Dupuytren'schen Kontraktur. *Brun's Beiträge für klinische Chirurgie*, **198**, 1.

MILLESI, H. (1965). Zur Pathogenese und Therapie der Dupuytren'schen Kontraktur. Eine Studie an Hand von mehr als 500 Fällen. *Ergebnisse der Chirurgie und Orthopädie*, **47**, 51.

MOORHEAD, J. J. (1956). Dating the Onset of Dupuytren's Contracture. *American Journal of Surgery*, **92**, 571.

MOSER, E. (1936). Einiges über die Dupuytrensche Fingerkontraktur. *Zentralblatt für Chirurgie*, **63**, 149.

NAUCK, E. TH. (1931). Die Wellung der Sehnenfasern, ihre Ursache und ihre fonktionelle Bedeutung. *Morphologisches Jahrbuch*, **68**, 79.

NEZELOF, C. & TUBIANA, R. (1958). La maladie de Dupuytren. Étude histologique. *Semaine des Hôpitaux de Paris*, **34**, 1102.

SHAW, H. M. (1951). The treatment of Dupuytren's contracture. *British Journal of Plastic Surgery*, **18**, 164–170.

SHAW, H. M. & EASTWOOD, D. S. (1965). Dupuytren's contracture. A selective approach to treatment. *British Journal of Plastic Surgery*, **18**, 164–170.

SKOOG, T. (1948). Dupuytren's contraction. *Acta chirurgica scandinavica*, **96**, suppl. 139.

SKOOG, T. (1967). Dupuytren's contracture: pathogenesis and surgical treatment. *Surgical Clinics of North America*, **47**, no. 2.

SNELL, J. (1971). Delayed primary split skin grafting for Dupuytren's contracture. In: *Transactions of the 5th Congress of the International Confederation of Plastic and Reconstructive Surgery, Melbourne 22–26th February 1971*.

SNYDER, C. C. (1957). Dupuytren's contracture. *Annals of Surgery*, **23**, 487.

STACK, H. G. (1967). Anatomy of fascia in web space. Handchirurgisches Symposium in Wein, 28–30th May 1967.

TIMOTHY, A. et al. (1956). Clinical aspects of D.C. *Journal of the International College of Surgeons*, **26**, 232.

THOMINE, J. (1965). Conjonctive d'enveloppe du doigt et squelette fibreux des commissures inter-digitales. *Annales de Chirurgie plastique*, **10**, 194–203.

TUBIANA, R. (1955). Prognosis and treatment of Dupuytren's contracture. *Journal of Bone and Joint Surgery*, **37A**, 1155.

TUBIANA, R. (1965). Le traitement selectif de la maladie de Dupuytren. *Revue de Chirurgie orthopédique et réparatrice de l'Appareil moteur*, **50**, 311–334.

WEBB-JONES, A. (1965). Dupuytren's contracture. The results of radical fasciectomy. *British Journal of Plastic Surgery*, **18**, 377–384.

ZACHARIAE, L. (1967). Extensive versus limited fasciectomy for Dupuytren's contracture. *Scandinavian Journal for Plastic and Reconstructive Surgery*, **1**, 150–153.

ZACHARIAE, L. (1969). Dupuytren's contracture. *Scandinavian Journal for Plastic and Reconstructive Surgery*, **3**, 145–149.

9. PROGNOSIS AS A GUIDE TO THE TIMING AND EXTENT OF SURGERY IN DUPUYTREN'S CONTRACTURE

J. T. Hueston

The selection of the best operation for each individual patient is one of the most interesting aspects of Dupuytren's contracture.

In this paper it is hoped to point out the prognostic basis for the selection of surgery in Dupuytren's contracture. This presumes two things:
1. There is no universal operation for Dupuytren's contracture.
2. That some assessment for prognosis is possible.

Prognosis is based on the natural history of Dupuytren's contracture which varies from patient to patient in porportion to the strength of the constitutional tendency or diathesis in each patient. Some factors to be considered in assessing the prognosis are:
(a) General factors; family history, age of onset, sex of patient, epilepsy and alcoholism.
(b) Local factors; distribution of lesions, ectopic deposits, rate of progress to date and the effects of previous surgery.

A *family history* indicates by its severity the likelihood of rapid progress but it is accepted that a negative family history is not to be taken literally because very few patients (apart from doctors) have accurate knowledge of the hands of elderly relatives.

The *age of onset* is often younger in patients with a positive family history and certainly the younger the age of onset the worse the prognosis because, not only is there a correspondingly longer life span for continued progress but the pathological process is usually more active and more diffuse in younger patients. Thus the condition requires more extensive surgery than in elderly patients, if the hand is to be restored to full working potential and recurrence is to be minimized.

The *sex* of the patient influences the prognosis because in women the onset is usually later and the progress slower but the incidence of postoperative interphalangeal joint stiffness is higher than in men. Because elderly women are usually better able to accommodate to the nuisance of finger deformity when it does occur, surgery is less often recommended in women.

Epilepsy and alcoholism enjoy a bad reputation in the prognostic assessment of Dupuytren's contracture for reasons which as yet are far from clear.

Distribution of lesions in the hands is almost infinitely variable, but whereas bands on the radial side of the hand can often be left unoperated because of the slow progress of first web space contraction and the very rare production of metacarpophalangeal and interphalangeal deformity of the thumb, lesions on the ulnar side of the hand frequently show rapid progress, perhaps because of the lesser stretching influence on these digits solely reserved for power gripping. Certainly involvement of A.D.M. in the little finger nodule requires urgent surgery if P.I.P. deformity is to be totally correctable, certainly before the onset of the D.I.P. hyperextension is associated with boutonniere type deformity. The interdigital band without palmar involvement has a poorer prognosis in that proximal interphalangeal deformity is frequently incompletely correctable and recurrence is common. Hence Wolfe graft replacement of skin is often to be considered in this lesion.

Bilateral lesions of any distribution are taken to mean a stronger diathesis but the plan of operation in each hand is usually decided on its own merits.

Ectopic deposits such as knuckle pads or plantar nodules are evidence of a stronger diathesis and therefore, taken in conjunction with other signs suggesting the likelihood of recurrence would be a factor in making the surgery more radical rather than less radical.

The progress to date of any patient is of course a good indication of the likely future progress, and therefore the type of surgery to be required. A short history with rapid progression of deformity requires urgent radical surgery. An elderly man showing no progress over several years need not be operated on at all.

Finally the *results of previous surgery* are a good indication of the reactive state of the patient's hand—and early recurrence from previous fasciectomy will suggest a more radical local operation, perhaps with skin replacement, while residual joint stiffness or, even worse, an intrinsic plus hand, should be a warning against intervention of any type unless it is absolutely essential.

Bearing these prognostic facts in mind, the advice to any particular patient may be (a) no surgery at present because of the absence of deformity and likelihood of very slow progress: but a review later is advised so that, if the lesion progresses, the optimum time for surgery can be chosen.

(b) Palmar fasciotomy to temporize in senile patients by lessening troublesome metacarpophalangeal deformity for their last few years.

(c) Local fasciectomy to remove the deforming mechanism and correct deformity, warning that, although metacarpophalangeal deformities are nearly always totally correctable, P.I.P. deformity is not always totally correctable.

(d) Limited fasciectomy is the commonest operation advised because most patients show only mild evidence of diathesis and it has the advantages of shorter morbidity. These patients are warned that extension elsewhere in the hand may later require further surgery (but since these hands are usually fully functional three weeks after operation it is not too great a burden to be anticipated again in 5–10 years time).

(e) *A radical palmar fasciectomy* with separate dissection of affected digits, is advised in young patients with multifocal palmar lesions and progressive metacarpophalangeal deformity. The slightly longer morbidity and the possibility of extension in unoperated areas requiring later surgery are pointed out to the patient.

(f) Radical local excision of both fascia and skin with *Wolfe graft replacement* is advised in those young patients with a strong diathesis evidenced by recurrence after previous surgery, or where by the rate of progress to date and the weight of predisposing factors such as epilepsy or alcoholism, a strong family history and ectopic deposits, it seems predictable that local recurrence will occur. Skin replacement has usually been reserved for such lesions in the ring and little fingers.

(g) *Amputation* is advised when uncorrectable interphalangeal deformity in the little finger is sufficient nuisance and has the advantage in elderly patients of a short convalescence.

In summary, the surgeon's advice to any patient with Dupuytren's contracture may take one of seven different forms, his decision being made after considering the factors likely to influence the prognosis in each particular patient. It is stressed that the results after surgery are as much decided by the type of patient as by the type of surgery.

10. OBSERVATIONS ON DUPUYTREN'S DISEASE

Patrick Clarkson

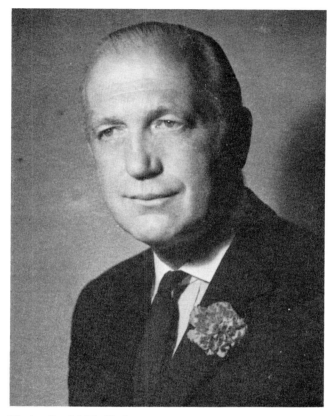

The late Patrick W. Clarkson.

In their article, Pulvertaft and Reid (1963) in their authoritative survey of British Hand Surgery state: 'It is humbling to reflect that although Dupuytren's disease has been known since the descriptions by Plater (1614), Astley Cooper (1822) and Guillaume Dupuytren (1832) the cause remains obscure and there is no general agreement as to the ideal method of surgical treatment. The accepted predisposing factors are age, sex, race and heredity.'

There is still doubt about the varying importance of all these factors. Clarkson and Pelly (1962) state that 'Baron Dupuytren, of Paris and Limoges, who lived in the first half of the nineteenth century is now seldom remembered except for his contribution to the "maladie de Dupuytren" and his classification of burns by their depth.' Conway (1954) has, however, reminded us of

what a dominant figure he was in his day, one of the true master surgeons of the century in which he lived and a man who made contributions over the whole field of surgery as it then was. The concern here is with his contribution to the surgery of the hand which can truly be called a permanent and original one, although he was historically preceded by Cooper (1822) and Cline (1808) in his recognition of the fascial origin of the disease and even in his suggestions for treatment; nor have his views on its aetiology which favour trauma as a precipitating or aggravating agent remained unchallenged.

It is interesting to note that the Baron's views on the fascial origin of the maladie have, in contrast to his views on aetiology, remained. His conservative views on surgical management have until recently remained largely unchanged; this contrasts with the challenges to his views on the role of trauma in aetiology, and for a time, on his extremely conservative views on the role of surgery in the treatment of the maladie. These conservative views on treatment prevail more now, but for a 25 year period in the middle of the twentieth century, much more radical surgical excisions were practised and advocated.

Hueston (1963) reminds us: 'The account given in the first chapter of Dupuytren's *Leçons de Clinque Chirurgicale* was not penned by the Baron Dupuytren himself but taken down as lecture notes at the Hotel Dieu and differs from the account published in *Lancet* of 1834.'

On the historical side, Hueston notes that Plater (1680) while describing the condition and its progress 'does not attempt an explanation of its cause or pathology' and that priority rests with Cline's lectures. However, the first written account is Cooper's 'brief but concise note in 1822'; the maladie is to be treated only when the thecae are not affected, 'as no operation or other means will succeed; but when the aponeurosis is the cause of the contraction and the contracted band is narrow, it may be with advantage divided by a pointed bistoury . . . followed by splintage.'

Hueston also notes that Goyrand (1834), a surgeon at the Hotel-Dieu at Aix, gave very precise details of the course and attachments of the bands involving the thumb in a man aged 72 years. The palmar aponeurosis was said to be normal and 'the fingers were held in flexion by newly formed fibrous cords, some of which passed from the palmar aponeurosis to insert distally

63

to the flexor tendon sheath or to the edges of the phalanges'.

Goyrand claimed, therefore, that Dupuytren had been in error to have attributed this condition to 'a retraction of the palmar aponeurosis', and goes on to add that, 'a traumatic basis for this retraction was unwarranted'.

AETIOLOGY

The accepted factors in aetiology, which are agreed by Pulvertaft and Reid, Hueston and Clarkson and Pelly, as well as many preceding authors, are age, race familial diathesis, and, to some extent, sex. Although the sex differential between male and female may be high in the younger age groups, Early (1962) and Gordon (1954) have shown that it is very much less in the older age groups.

The disease is virtually unknown in the first decade, and the author has seen only two cases in the second decade. The most common age of onset is in the fifth decade when it may be present in 2–3 per cent of the adult population. It then increases markedly with each decade of life when it may reach 40 per cent in the eighties (Hueston, 1963).

Graubard (1954) claims that development of Dupuytren is dependent upon two factors: (1) an inherited predisposition, indicated by genetic study of the Rh factor, and (2) the exposure of predisposed persons to specific trauma. The author believes this to be a rational approach. Hueston states that Graubard is not supported by the studies of Verso of the Australian Red Cross which showed that in 50 cases there were only six with group Rh1 RH2 which is the normal distribution.

Pulvertaft and Reid (1963) assess the family history as '30 per cent of cases, but it is manifestly difficult to arrive at an accurate figure'; Skoog (1948) gave it as 44 per cent.

RACE

During the last 150 years it has been the common observation of nearly all writers on this disease that it is much more common in non-pigmented—particularly Anglo-Saxon skins—than in pigmented skins. It is notably more common in white Americans than coloured Americans and virtually unknown in Chinese and the Formosans (Clarkson and Pelly, 1962).

Hueston states: 'Racial or ethnic or even familial predisposition to certain diseases is now recognized and the proclivity of identical twins for identical disease is perhaps the strongest example of such an association.''

The point must be made in discussing incidence in coloured Africans that the maladie must be distinguished from the not uncommon condition of post-framboesial palmar fibrosis (Clarkson and Pelly, 1962).

RELATION TO TRAUMA

The significance attached to trauma has varied throughout the known history of the disease. Baron Dupuytren considered the chronic trauma was a factor in his coachman. For 70 to 80 years the authoritative view, represented by Bunnell, has been that trauma was neither a precipitating nor an aggravating agent.

In a survey by Clarkson (1961) of numerous authorities, he found that most oppose the view that a direct relationship exists between trauma and the presence of the disease, but some of the authorities he contacted, especially Rank and James, quoted highly suggestive evidence that trauma to the medial side of the palm which had been followed by fixation of the digits in flexion, might have a very real causal relationship to the precipitation or aggravation of the disease. Clarkson therefore concluded that a single trauma, severe or otherwise, can cause the onset of the disease in a predisposed person. He also refers to the strong relationship between neurological disease or damage—cerebral, spinal, or ulnar nerve—with the onset and progress of contracture of the medial digits associated with palmar nodules.

On the other hand, many historic studies including those of Early (1962), Herzog (1951) and Hueston (1963) failed, in large groups, to show any occupational connection with chronic trauma; but Lund (1941) and Graubard (1954) (quoted by Hueston, 1963) claim that there is a significantly high incidence of Dupuytren's disease among brewery works and alcoholics.

Skoog (1948) is, of course, the classic authority in support of the connection between chronic trauma and the incidence of the disease; he states that 'there is an increased frequency amongst persons in occupations with considerable mechanical strain on the hands'.

PATHOLOGY

Three stages can be recognized in the pathological course of the disease: (1) the nodule; (2) the early or reversible flexion contracture; (3) the late or irreversible contracture.

In stage (1) the palmar nodule may be the only manifestation of the disease. No contracture may be present at this point.

Hueston (1963) considers that 'in most patients the start is a palmar nodule but in a few a short interphalangeal band deformity occurs. In 10 per cent of cases nodules are found in relation to the thumb'.

MacCallum and Hueston (1962) give new support to an old concept. This view they support with very considerable clinical and pathological evidence. It is that the nodule lies in the fibrous fatty layer, that is, it originates superficial to the palmar fascia which it involves secondarily as it does the skin. 'No definite instance has been observed of a palmar nodule disappearing although this has been reported by careful observers including Gordon (1948) and Iselin (1954).'

In stage (1) the palmar nodule can be the only manifestation of the disease. No contracture may be present, and none may ever occur, the disease remaining arrested at this point (Clarkson and Pelly, 1962).

Stages (2) and (3)

Nodules in the distal palm or overlying the proximal phalanx of the digit, cause flexion contracture at the metacarpophalangeal joints; this latter contracture is associated with hyperextension of the distal interphalangeal joint due to traction effect on the lateral extensor slips. The classical flexion contracture of Dupuytren's disease is therefore associated with hyperextension deformity of the terminal digital joint.

Flexion contracture most commonly involves the ring finger (43 per cent of cases); the little finger is the next most commonly involved (34 per cent of cases). Contracture of the nodule is the causal agent. The rate at which flexion contracture follows is dependent in part on age, and in part on innate individual variation. In the second and third decades, progress may be so rapid that the tip of the affected finger touches the palm in 3 months (Clarkson and Pelly, 1962).

A period of 3 to 5 years in the fifth decade and after would be considered rapid progress of the disease. Variability in the rate of progress is the outstanding clinical feature and must be dominant in the mind of the surgeon determining individual treatment (Clarkson, 1963).

Hueston's views on pathology and natural history must be quoted:

The palmar nodule may remain stationary for decades ... confluence of adjacent foci in the central palm may produce a raised plaque across which the flexor creases pass deeply and over which the epidermis and dermis become fixed. ... An early band is usually better developed proximal to the nodule and distally is still opaque with fat loculi incorporated in its surface. Although continuous with the aponeurosis, the band stands forward several millimetres and lies close beneath the skin.

Discrete dense tendinous bands continuous with the distal end of a thickened intertendinous septum are sometimes found passing through the neck of the metacarpal to the proximal phalanx grossly displacing the neurovascular bundle and maintaining a flexion deformity after excision of the principal pretendinous band ... The role of work hypertrophy in the production of the bands, which has been propounded by Luck (1959) is supported by the atrophy of the band when the tension is relieved by fasiotomy.'

Hueston (1963) further states:

'Despite meticulous excision of aponeurosis and abnormal tissue a recurrence of Dupuytren's tissue

is common in those patients who required operation while the disease was rapidly progressing and particularly if they have a strong family history. Recurrences in the finger require secondary excision more often than those in the palm and at operation have macroscopic features strikingly similar to a virgin case. These nodules or recurrent Dupuytren's tissue indicate that, as they could no longer have arisen from any pre-existing anatomical fascial bands, they must have developed from the normal fibrofatty tissue remaining in the region.'

ASSOCIATED LESIONS

The lesions to be discussed are those of: (1) knuckle pads; (2) the foot; (3) the penis.

Knuckle pads. Knuckle pads over the proximal interphalangeal joints are common in Dupuytren's disease, but the exact incidence is unknown. McIndoe (1958) said that if a patient had knuckle pads he either had or would eventually develop Dupuytren's disease in the palm of the hand. Most surgeons would agree with this opinion.

Foot lesion. The lesion in the foot commonly starts as a symptomless lump of the subcutaneous tissue high on the instep and attached to the plantar fascia. It generally starts spontaneously but the author has seen a case in a boy which followed rupture of the plantar fascia by a fall on his feet on to a concrete surface from a considerable height, and which was immediately followed by a haematoma.

The condition is commonly described as symptomless and not warranting operation. It is the author's experience that such nodules are commonly tender to pressure and considerably limit the activities of energetic people. He has also seen a case of bilateral, painful nodules on the inner sides of each big toe with associated paraesthesia of the digital nerves to them in feet with large plantar nodules.

Peyronie's disease. The association of Peyronie's disease or penile squint with Dupuytren's disease has often been noted, but the actual incidence is speculative. Hueston (1963) found this lesion present in only 6 out of 224 patients with Dupuytren's disease. In 10 patients seen with Peyronie's disease by the same author, 4 had Dupuytren's disease.

Skoog (1948) found only 7 out of 207 epileptics with penile plaques. Hueston notes:

'The degree of chordee and associated pain on erection varies according to the site of the plaque, being worse with the more distal lesions. ... The histological structure is similar to that of knuckle pads, and, although statistically the incidence of association between these penile lesions and Dupuytren's contracture is less obvious than with knuckle pads or plantar lesions, it is still possible to regard them as related and reflecting another facet of the diathesis we are considering.'

II. *MYSTERIOUS ASPECTS OF DUPUYTREN'S CONTRACTURE*

Marc Iselin

Dupuytren's contracture is a mysterious disease in that it is not possible for us to explain its nature or behaviour on the basis of currently accepted lines of thought. Likewise the only treatment that we have to combat it is surgery of the most simple nature, namely to cut the tight bands and to excise the abnormal areas.

It is worthwhile therefore to ask a series of questions which for the moment we are not able to answer.

1. Why should this essentially benign lesion spread by invasion of the surrounding tissues in the nature of a malignant tumour and not by expansion as would any other benign tumour?

2. Why should this lesion, so often referred to as contraction of the palmar aponeurosis, invade the fingers in various forms and thus produce the most serious disabilities from the disease and certainly introduce the most difficult operative requirements— particularly as there is no palmar aponeurosis in the digits?

3. Why should the palmar aponeurosis be involved more often in certain spots and less in others?

4. Why should the onset of this condition most often be quite sudden? A nodule which had not been present the day before is obvious the following morning.

5. Why should the natural history of this condition be so unpredictable? It may stay the same for some years or progressively increase; disappear or reappear in the same spot; become suddenly contracted and pull the fingers down into flexion, when for several years it has not touched them?

6. Why should even the most straightforward post-operative course suddenly be interrupted by swelling of the hand and Sudek's atrophy of an apparently psychosomatic origin?

7. Why should the albumin:globulin ratio also show unpredictable variation, sometimes above and sometimes below normal? These variations seem to play a significant role in the healing process.

We will consider now the surgical implications of these mysterious aspects in evolving a theory of causation which, although purely intellectual, may stimulate further scientific studies in order to answer these questions.

1. EXTENSION BY INVASION

It has been constantly observed by all surgeons that the lesions present usually as firm fibrous masses, some in the form of bands and others as plaques; but there is no plane of cleavage and in order to dissect them it is necessary to cut along their macroscopic edges at the apparent margin of healthy tissue. It is particularly important to cut the points of fixation to the skin which is invaded and often retracted. Ablation of the lesions and correction of the deformities leaves an empty space which is not filled in by the adjacent tissues as would be the case after removal of a benign tumour. The space remains open, filled with blood clot which leads on to scar tissue, the behaviour of which affects the final outcome. Thus if it heals well the hand remains supple and normal, which happily is in the majority of cases. But if healing produces a tendency to contracture, both the skin and the fingers are pulled on anew ending up with what we call a 'false recurrence'. On secondary operation this fibrous tissue is clearly seen as a layer of diffuse scar of variable thickness as it is excised, and histologically it proves to be pure scar with nothing in common with the original tissue of the Dupuytren's contracture.

2. INVASION OF THE FINGERS

Invasion of the fingers is the most serious factor in this disease since it leads to flexion of the phalanges which is the basis of our classification into 4 degrees. The actual pathological lesions have the same glistening pearly appearance as in the palm but their distribution is extremely variable.

They may present as ill-defined bands or more often as nodules but in any case they can displace the digital nerves.

Relation between the lesions and the digital nerves:

All the operative difficulties in Dupuytren's contracture are associated with the dissection of the digital nerves which, although not completely surrounded, are closely intermingled and more or less adherent to the abnormal tissue. Unhappy experience has shown that even the most careful operator is always in danger of dividing a nerve, sometimes in the palm but more often in the fingers, because they are displaced unpredictably by the development of these fibrous areas— this displacement is most unpredictable in that area where the nerves pass from the palm into the fingers at the level of the web spaces.

Surgical division of a nerve is always to be taken seriously because of the trophic disturbances which it may initiate. If it is recognized it should be repaired immediately. In almost every case of recurrence that we have operated on, one or more nerves have been found to have been cut and not repaired.

IN THE PALM

The attachment of the palmar aponeurosis and the intertendinous septa prevents any serious displacement of the relationship of the nerves from the subaponeurotic plane where they lie in the intertendinous septa. The only abnormality may be when they become too close and adhere to the deep aspect of the aponeurosis.

AT THE LEVEL OF THE WEB SPACE

The relationship of the nerves at this level are of two types:

(a) Normal, where the nerve stays under the superficial aponeurosis and within the interosseous septum.

(b) Abnormal and dangerous, where the nerve is found to lie superficial to the fibrous structures because of infiltration of the deeper extension of the palmar aponeurosis crossing the nerve obliquely. This pushes the nerve out of place and presents it under the skin ready to be cut by the scalpel if the surgeon is not expecting it in this situation. The nerve is thus found more lateral to the main fibrous infiltration in the palm and in line with it at the base of the fingers but all these normal relations can be changed and the nerve lie superficial to the aponeurosis than progressively within it and finally behind it. A surgeon cannot be too much on guard for these abnormalities, the fear of which is one of the greatest arguments in favour of incisions which generously expose this dangerous region.

IN THE FINGERS

According to whether the nodules have developed in the palmar aponeurosis or the deeper septum, so the relations of the nerves vary and we can distinguish three main variations.

Type 1—the nerve stays in its normal course under the aponeurosis along the lateral side of the finger and if a nodule invades the deep septum this is superficial and parallel to the nerve—nevertheless either the nodule itself or an expansion from it passing to the lateral side of the middle phalanx may cross in front of the nerve. Under this arcade the nerve is free in its areolar sheath but it is these cases in which the nerve can sometimes be said literally to pass through the nodule if it expands sufficiently in a dorsal direction.

Type 2—the nerve is pushed towards the midline of the finger by a nodule which has developed almost solely from the superficial aponeurosis and by virtue of its oblique direction crosses the nerve either above or below, about the level of the web space. However,

at the level of the middle phalanx the nerve returns to its normal place along the lateral border of the finger, whether it has gone around the nodule either in front or behind as described in the previous type.

Type 3—the nerve is similarly pushed towards the midline of the finger by a nodule which is going to insert on the side of the proximal phalanx but which stays under

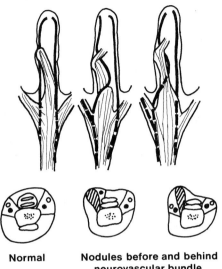

**Normal   Nodules before and behind
                          neurovascular bundle**

Figure 11.1

it when it crosses it the first time at the level of the web space, only to be recrossed more distally by it on a more superficial plane. There is thus a point where the nerve is directly subcutaneous without anything to give warning of this state of affairs and of course it can be divided as soon as the skin is incised.

These abnormal relationships account for nerve injuries without the nerves being seen, for it is literally in danger from the skin incision.

3. UNPREDICTABILITY OF LESIONS —THEIR APPEARANCE, GROWTH AND ULTIMATE DISAPPEARANCE

We can not predict these aspects. When we understand the cause of this disease then we will be in the position to consider prevention and non-surgical cure.

At present we can only resort to theories but these observations allow us to propose operative indications and some choice of the appropriate procedures. As far as theories are concerned the only one which seems to us to explain these otherwise inexplicable observations is that involving polymerization of the connective tissues under certain unknown influences which affect not only the palmar aponeurosis but also the tiniest fibrous strands of the fingers as well as the tendons and interosseous muscles. The disappearance of nodules could then be explained on the basis of depolymerization for it is well known that connective tissues can be depolymerized much the same as plastic material. So far we have not found a scientist who will work on this theory but this is worthy of further study, which is unfortunately beyond the capacity of a mere surgeon.

Without, however, being able to resolve these curious facts they do themselves have considerable practical surgical importance. The abnormal anatomy created by the disease is more important to us than the normal anatomy of the hand and in particular the operative possibilities of displaced nerves and invasion of tendons carry considerable danger in the first case and the need to reconsider the exposure of the lesions in particular in the more severely flexed fingers.

THE SURGICAL EXPOSURE OF CERTAIN DIGITAL LESIONS

Generally the digital lesions are exposed from the volar aspect in the first and second degrees of flexion and from the dorsal aspect from the third and fourth degrees of more severe flexion and these latter are what interest us in this context.

The third degree has flexion of the terminal phalanx more than the proximal two phalanges and moreover the band holding this terminal phalanx in flexion is generally small, flat and very laterally placed. A search for this from a volar exposure is likely to be unsuccessful. Exposure by the dorsal approach, however, presents it immediately and both its recognition and removal can be done with the greatest safety while skin closure is easy and scar retraction is no problem at this level.

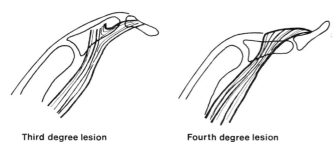

Third degree lesion   **Fourth degree lesion**

Figure 11.2

In the same way for the fourth stage when the fibrous mass holding the proximal phalanges in flexion follows the interosseous expansion dorsally and produces contracture of the extensor apparatus with resultant hyperextension. Only the dorsal exposure allows clarification of the precise nature of the lesions and adequate successful treatment.

Finally it is worth stressing that the third and fourth degree often requires that the flexion deformity be corrected in two stages—the first by volar approach to clear the palmar lesions as far as the middle phalanx, and then a second stage after healing and rehabilitation

to correct the terminal joint deformity using the dorsal approach.

4. PSYCHOLOGICAL FACTORS IN THE CAUSATION OF POSTOPERATIVE SWELLING AND STIFFNESS

It is difficult to assess the incidence of these serious postoperative complications of oedema and joint stiffness as they are so differently reported (9 of 195 by Thomine; 50 per cent by Boyes).

Several factors have rightly been blamed. Tight bandages are a serious error but one which can be corrected on the next day by loosening the bandages and evaluating the hand—and certainly we never allow a complete plaster to be applied after surgery for Dupuytren's contracture.

Skin necrosis and infection—the process here is not altogether clear for oedema can follow apparently normal healing and even appear as late as two or three weeks after surgery, even of such a minor extent as subcutaneous fasciotomy.

Howard has stated quite strongly that there is only one major problem in the surgery of Dupuytren's contracture, that is the prevention of postoperative joint stiffness and its treatment if it should appear. While technique is important in lessening the incidence there is no doubt that stiffness can appear without relation to the type of incision, the occurrence of haematoma or of cutaneous skin loss.

It would appear to us to be an angioneurotic oedema arising from local reflexes controlling the trophicity of the tissues and controlled by psychological factors as well. It is common in nervous, anxious and difficult patients and can be prevented and materially assisted in its treatment by tranquillizers or antidepressives according to the case. An osteo-articular dystrophy syndrome is called 'osteoporosis' in France because of the radiological picture, the Germans call it 'Sudek's atrophy' and the Scandinavians merely 'dystrophy' but whatever its name it is worthwhile quickly running over those aspects which seem important in unravelling this problem.

1. The oedema is not merely superficial but occurs deeply as well, even involving the bone and the so-called 'osteoporosis' is in fact best regarded as an oedema of the bone.

2. The clinical oedema provides the link between the functional and the organic because, while it arises from a purely physiological disturbance of the permeability of the capillaries, it is on the other hand the origin of the subsequent sclerosis and contractions.

3. The articular reflexes were stressed by Leriche as the origin of pain and the secondary vasomotor effect would account for the origin of this oedema.

4. The persistence of these reflexes is explicable on the basis of conditioned patterns involving the cerebral motor areas of the joints as well as the psyche and pain sensory areas, which set up a continuing self-stimulating cycle.

A psychosomatic origin would thus seem to explain the onset of the osteoarthritic dystrophy syndrome after Dupuytren's contracture and certainly this has been confirmed by the paper by Ehlers and Zachariae from Copenhagen.

Certainly a psychiatric assessment of patients before operation may help in this management and particularly with the psycholeptic postoperative therapy which seems in our hands to have greatly diminished the occurrence of postoperative swelling and stiffness.

5. ABNORMALITIES OF GLOBULIN:ALBUMIN RATIO

We recognize two disturbances of protein metabolism in these patients namely hypoproteinaemia in which the total proteins are lowered and dysproteinaemia in which the albumin:globulin ratio is disturbed.

The total protein level is important in the healing process which will be disturbed by anything which causes hypoproteinaemia. It is more difficult still to correct disturbances of the albumin:globulin ratio but in a hyperanabolic state when the ratio is below 1:5 a catabolic hormone such as cortisone could be used and in a hypo-anabolic state when the ratio is above 1:5 some anabolic hormone such as testosterone may be tried. Thus it is necessary to make these protein estimations before operation and we have been astonished at the variety of levels which have been encountered without anything in the patient's general condition to have suggested these abnormalities in their metabolism. It has even been found that when the albumin:globulin ratio was normal before the operation it became abnormal in the first few postoperative days, showing the need to repeat these tests if the postoperative course is not satisfactory, and if an abnormality is detected to proceed with its correction at once.

From all this it is clear that few other diseases show so many mysteries, that is to say so many obvious facts impossible as yet to explain. The facts are important to us as surgeons and if we are aware of them and think along the lines that have been indicated in this paper we can help in the assessment of operative indications and both pre and postoperative care. It is for the scientist ultimately to explain the details of these mechanisms.

REFERENCES

EHLERS, H. & ZACHARIAE, L. (1964). Mentality and dystrophy. *Acta orthopaedica scandinavica*, **34,** 109–113.

GOSSET, J. (1964). Les résultats de l'aponévrectomie large dans la maladie de Dupuytren. *Mémoires de l'Academie de Chirurgie*, **90,** 756–759.

HOWARD, L. D. (1959). Dupuytren's contracture, a guide to management. *Clinical Orthopedics*, **15** (12), 118–126.

ISELIN, F. (1965). Les appareils de correction et de rééducation en chirurgie de la main. *Journal de Chirurgie (Paris)*, **89,** 207–220.

ISELIN, M. & ISELIN, F. (1965). Types of Z plasty and their technical determination. *Journal of the International College of Surgeons*, **43,** 276–286.

ISELIN, M. & ISELIN, F. (1966). Complications post-opératoires dans la maladie de Dupuytren. *Mémoires de l'Academie de Chirurgie*, **92,** 240–246.

ISELIN, M. & ISELIN, F. (1967). *Traite de Chirurgie de la Main*. Paris: Flammarion.

JAMES, J. I. P. & TUBIANA, R. (1952). La maladie de Dupuytren (Rapport de la XXVIIᵉ Reunion de la Societe Française d'Orthopédie et Traumatologie. In *Revue de Chirurgie orthopédique et réparatrice de l'Appareil moteur*, **38,** 352–406.

PARRINI, L. & BRUNELLI, G. (1965). La maladie de Dupuytren. *Rapport au IIIᵉ Congres de la Societe Italienne de Chirurgie de la Main, Modene*.

PEACOCK, E. E. (1964). Dupuytren's contracture. *Reconstructive Plastic Surgery* (edited by J. M. Converse), pp. 1728–1739. Philadelphia: Saunders.

THOMINE, J. M. (1964). Contribution a l'étude de la maladie de Dupuytren et de son traitement chirurgical. Thesis, Paris.

TUBIANA, R. (1964). Le traitement sélectif de la maladie de Dupuytren. *Revue de Chirurgie orthopédique et réparatrice de l'Appareil moteur*, **50,** 331–334.

12. THE PRINCIPLES OF SURGICAL TREATMENT OF DUPUYTREN'S CONTRACTURE

Raoul Tubiana

Considerations of the treatment of Dupuytren's contracture have always been centred around the two types of operation advocated for its treatment—wide excision aimed at prophylaxis and limited excision. One might say that Dupuytren practised only fasciotomies but the surgery of this condition had advanced sufficiently by the beginning of this century that Lexer, disappointed by the poor results of limited surgery, was advocating an extended excision both of the aponeurosis and of the overlying skin and subcutaneous tissue. The frequency and the severity of complications after extensive surgery, however, has caused a return to more limited surgical intervention.

Arguments are advanced by those advocating either extensive or limited surgery and have used nearly every aspect of the disease to support their surgical bias, ranging from aetiological aspects through pathology and clinical features to the final results of therapy.

In this paper I would first like to consider certain controversial ideas such as the exact site of origin of the pathological process, the prophylactic value of fasciectomy, the basis of the surgical complications and the management of the skin—and then by way of conclusion to present the data on which our present lines of management are based.

Before setting out to discuss the relative values of particular operations proposed for Dupuytren's contracture it is essential to define these operations more precisely. Most of the confusion has arisen in this regard because of the use of terms which sound very similar, and the different surgeons appearing to advocate different operations may in fact be overlapping these fields of definitions which must be made more precise.

Fasciotomy is the most limited of all these operations and can be either open or subcutaneous.

While it is quite common for a fasciotomy to be carried out in the palm it carries a greater risk. The combination of a limited open operation in the finger, with limited resection of tissue plus fasciotomy in the palm can be a useful combination.

Nodulectomy advocated by Luck, but confined to the excision merely of the nodule itself, which from his concept of the disease constitutes the active area and allows him to leave behind the bands which are regarded by him as secondary to the tension produced by the nodule, and subsequent involution is expected.

Simple excision of the abnormal tissue in Dupuytren's contracture without particular dissection and resection of recognized fascial planes is less than a fasciectomy and implies the leaving behind of macroscopically uninvolved fascial structures in the region. It may be that complete or partial excision of the diseased tissue, for instance the nodulectomy is 'partial'.

Fasciectomies are essentially different from the simple excisions because, as the name implies, they are planned as a systematic excision of the anatomical fascial pattern along with the diseased regions and clearly includes areas which are macroscopically normal. In practice the extent of these fasciectomies varies in three dimensions both in a transverse direction, longitudinally, and in depth, which may include even the overlying skin.

In the transverse direction the fasciectomy for Dupuytren's contracture is theoretically aimed at removal of the superficial palmar aponeurosis and its extensions. Thus it can be considered 'complete transversely' when the excision of the fascia includes the whole pattern extending with its four rays of the superficial palmar aponeurosis. It is incomplete transversely or 'partial' when it is confined to the excision only of certain palmar rays usually on the medial side of the palm. It can be regarded as 'extensive' when more than the superficial palmar aponeurosis is excised and the specimen includes the fascia of both the thenar and hypothenar eminences.

In the longitudinal direction the fasciectomy commences usually fairly proximal in the palm, usually just proximal to the superficial palmar arch. Distally at the digital level, only the fingers with macroscopic lesions are operated upon. It is not a clearcut anatomical dissection of the fascia but only of the abnormal tissue.

In depth fasciectomy can be regarded as 'complete' only if it extends from the deep aspect of the palmar aponeurosis to the overlying skin which is resected with it. There are innumerable fascial fibres attaching to the deep aspect of the dermis particularly in the distal part of the palm and within the digits.

We would stress that the terms 'total' or 'radical' fasciectomy should never be used because it is a practical impossibility.

THE SITE OF ORIGIN OF THE LESIONS

MACROSCOPIC ANATOMY

Until the last few years it was generally accepted that the condition known as Dupuytren's contracture was a disease of the superficial palmar aponeurosis.

John Hueston had been struck by the importance and the extent of involvement of the fibrofatty tissue between the skin and the palmar aponeurosis and considered this layer to be not only the site of origin of the original disease but also that of recurrence. This point of view has led to palmar fasciectomy being considered no longer as the sole procedure to be adopted in curing and preventing this condition and has led to a more selective excision of the involved tissues instead of the previous routine extensive fasciectomy.

This theory has stimulated us to try to determine if the pathological process corresponds to the normal outline of the palmar aponeurosis and the digital fascia. One can certainly say that the severity and frequency of the fibroplastic lesions does not correspond precisely with the significant normal fascial structures. Thus the lesions of Dupuytren's contracture most commonly arise in the distal region of the palm but at this level the fascial structures are relatively slight and the longitudinal pretendinous bands tend to be lost on the deep aspect of the skin and the paratendinous septa are represented by little more than very fine and slender prolongations behind the neurovascular bundles as they pass to the fingers. It is therefore surprising and significant to realize that this region of the palm which is so poor in fascial and aponeurotic fibres is nevertheless among the areas most severely invaded by the contracting fibroplastic tissue of Dupuytren's contracture. It may be relevant that this area is also where the fibres of the aponeurosis have more dermal insertions than elsewhere.

This zone lies between the two fascial components of the palmar aponeurosis namely the superficial transverse ligament proximally which Skoog has noted as only rarely involved and the natatory ligament in the web space which on the contrary is very often involved.

Nevertheless despite the very irregular distribution of the pathological fibroplastic lesions it should not be concluded that these are without any relation whatsoever to the normal outline of the aponeurosis which it seems to follow in most cases. In the fingers particularly the displacements of the neurovascular bundle from its normal course is usually explicable by selective thickening from involvement of specific portions of the fascial envelope of the front of the finger. Sometimes the neurovascular bundle retains its normal relationship to the fibrous supporting structures on the front of the finger despite the degree of thickening in these structures and dissection is not very difficult—thus at the base of the finger the natatory ligament is superficial and sends fibres to reinforce the digital fascia, in particular the retrovascular band which passes at first anterior then medial, and finally posterior to the neurovascular bundle. At the level of the P.I.P. joint the deep layer of the digital fascia normally becomes attached to the

fibrous flexor sheath, having been separated from the side of the proximal phalanx by a plane of cleavage. Whatever the course of the band in the neurovascular bundle up to this level, the aponeurosis becomes attached deeply to the fibrous flexor sheath, leaving the neurovascular bundle to run superficially. It is at this level that the neurovascular bundle is most exposed to injury because it can quite suddenly be lifted forwards by a nodule in the deep plane of the normal digital fascia.

At the base of the little finger, superficial to the medial collateral neurovascular bundle of this finger there is often a nodule of variable thickness which fuses both with the fascia of the finger and with the hypothenar fascia. The neurovascular bundle is thus to be found between these two fibrous structures.

MICROSCOPIC ANATOMY

Histology offers little in elucidating the precise site of origin of the pathological process. These changes arise at first on the anterior aspect of the palmar aponeurosis and their progression is usually superficial along the lines of the fibrous strands passing into the dermis—but it would be presuming rather too much to conclude that involvement of the palmar aponeurosis is purely a secondary process. Nezelof considers that the changes in the fatty tissue superficial to the aponeurosis are more secondary than primary in the fibroplastic process. Millesi goes further and insists that the hyperplastic process never commences independently of the fascia but always in collagen fibres which have lost their normal appearance.

Jean Gosset proposes a clever compromise between the conflicting views when he attributes the origin of the fascial bands to specific aponeurotic lesions, but the clinically important nodule can be attributed to the process having arisen within the fibrofatty subcutaneous tissue. This ingenious distinction remains as yet to be proven.

We are forced to conclude from all these discussions that Dupuytren's contracture arises from a fibroplastic process which follows at least in part the outline of the palmar and digital fascial structures but also that this process is not confined purely to the aponeurosis.

This new notion must be taken into account when planning the treatment of this condition.

PROPHYLACTIC VALUE OF FASCIECTOMY

If we are to discuss the prophylactic value of a fasciectomy we must first distinguish true recurrences arising within the operative field from extensions arising in unoperated areas—although who can be certain of total excision of the aponeurosis in any particular field? Histologically there is little to distinguish because both recurrences and extensions are histologically much closer to the typical pattern of Dupuytren's contracture than to scar tissue.

'Total' or 'radical' fasciectomies have been planned to prevent extension of the disease elsewhere in the hand. This concept now seems to be untenable particularly as it is never possible to remove routinely the digital fascia from the normal fingers.

All the arguments about fasciectomy are therefore centred on the extent of the palmar fasciectomy whereas most recurrences and extensions occur in the fingers. The prophylactic value of palmar fasciectomy can not therefore, even when most optimistically supported, affect the areas where the subsequent appearance of lesions is most frequently observed. Prophylactic palmar aponeurosis can therefore only be concerned with preventing palmar extensions—it cannot prevent digital extensions—it does not prevent true palmar recurrences from arising in the area thus subjected to fasciectomy. Moreover it is possible as Hueston has suggested that recurrences develop not only from the remaining fascial elements but also from the other connective tissue elements becoming involved, namely the dermis and the subcutaneous fibrofatty tissue.

Recurrences also seem to be particularly likely to occur when certain general factors capable of influencing the development of the condition are more stongly present in some patients than others—the Dupuytren's diathesis.

These predisposing factors in the diathesis are a strong family history, the onset of the disease under 40 years, epilepsy and alcoholism, distribution of lesions particularly in the little finger and the association of ectopic lesions such as knuckle pads, plantar lesions and Peyronie's disease.

Excision either extensive of limited cannot stop the development of a generalized disease but nevertheless the percentage of recurrence must depend on the amount of tissue left behind which may be susceptible to the process.

Certainly the statistics of Millesi and Shaw show that there is a far higher recurrence rate after partial than after extensive fasciectomy.

If Hueston is correct—and our experience has agreed with his—when he says that recurrences and extensions occur most frequently in the two years after fasciectomy, then the natural history of the disease has not been arrested by the surgery. We have, like others, also seen of course a number of recurrences and extensions 5 to 10 years after fasciectomy.

The study of a series of McIndoe's cases operated by radical fasciectomy and followed up more than 11 years later by Hakstian is important in this regard. A general slow deterioration of hand function was found and about half the operated hands showed some evidence of progression of the disease with two-thirds of these requiring a secondary operation.

While we can recognize a set of circumstances or 'diathesis' favourable to the development and progression of lesions and recurrences there is on the other hand an opposite state of affairs where we can produce some regression of the fibroplastic lesions.

Occasionally spontaneously at the onset of the disease a nodule can shrink and get softer. Later in the disease a traumatic rupture of a longitudinal band can be seen to be followed by shrinkage of the fibroplastic nodule—much the same as can be observed after simple fasciotomy or a limited fasciectomy whose main effect has been to eliminate the longitudinal tension acting on the nodule. This behaviour of the fibrous tissue in Dupuytren's contracture is obviously comparable to that of hypertrophic scar tissue. Although this behaviour is far too unpredictable to be recommended in all cases it is enough to make one sceptical of the prophylactic value of total fasciectomy.

COMPLICATIONS OF FASCIECTOMY

One of the arguments often put forward by the advocates of limited surgery is the higher incidence of complications after extensive surgery. With Thomine we reviewed the postoperative complications of 195 extensive fasciectomies operated at the orthopaedic clinic of Cochin Hospital according to McIndoe's technique using a transverse palmar incision. Carried out between 1952 and 1962 this series does not represent the results of one single surgeon but of a group of surgeons of varying degree of experience.

Postoperative Oedema by itself without any other complication was taken to represent a personal reaction on the part of the patient to surgical trauma and occurred nine times. Three patients showed permanent stiffness with loss of flexion of all fingers.

Haematoma was the most common and the most serious of the postoperative complications of extensive fasciectomy. Despite careful haemostasis there were 31 palmar haematomas (16 per cent of operations) and 12 of these resulted in significant limitation of joint movement. A simple compression dressing was found to be insufficient to prevent haematomas because 21 haematomas occurred in the 85 hands when this alone was used. Controlled hypotension was used in 34 cases where the cardiovascular state allowed it and only 2 haematomas occurred when this was combined with pressure dressing. A dorsal plaster slab keeping the wrist in extension and the M.P. joints in slight flexion for ten days was found to produce an additional improvement and when used 20 times along with compression no haematoma occurred. We combine these three measures and now routinely at the end of operation use suction drainage for 48 hours.

Separation of the palmar incision was the commonest complication after haematoma and is attributed to the combination of mechanical traction on the wound and poor blood supply of the dissected palmar skin flaps. This occurred 20 times with 5 leaving permanent postoperative joint stiffness.

Necrosis of the palmar skin is rare after a single transverse incision (5 per cent of cases) but the incidence rose to 20 per cent in those cases where an L-shaped incision and elevation of a central palmar flap had been used. We therefore avoid all forms of angular flap design in the centre of the palm because of the poor blood supply and the poor elasticity of the skin in that area because we have been struck by the way in which purely palmar complications are able to disturb the hand as a whole and even leave permanent stiffness in previously quite normal fingers.

Skin problems in the fingers seem to be less serious and any permanent disability to be confined only to the involved finger. In 49 cases no healing problem was encountered following a simple lateral incision ending diagonally across the proximal phalanx whereas 4 out of 16 L-shaped digital incisions produced these complications.

The midline digital incision rearranged with Z-plasty was most used and showed about 10 per cent of complications (12 out of 123 cases) but the permanent disability was slight from these complications.

Division of digital nerves occurred in 15 cases.

Three factors seemed to have been important in determining the incidence of these postoperative complications. While the extent of the fasciectomy may be an important factor, the experience of the surgeon was obviously significant because the percentage of haematomas was only half as high and the incidence of skin necrosis and digital nerve division only one-third as high in the cases of the senior surgeons compared with those of the junior surgeons.

The third very important factor in the production of complications was the management of the overlying skin during the different forms of fasciectomy.

MANAGEMENT OF THE SKIN

In the light of present concepts of Dupuytren's contracture it would seem that an undue emphasis has been placed on the purely fascial and aponeurotic aspects of the disease and has tended to make surgeons overlook the importance of the management of the overlying skin. There is no doubt that the management of the skin both in exposing the lesions and in closing the wounds has an overriding influence both on the progress of the operation itself and on the postoperative course.

Surgical exposure must be capable of adaption to each case and to give only adequate exposure of both palmar and digital lesions but to allow rapid and uneventful healing. We have found that a high incidence of the complications of fasciectomy were due to badly selected incisions for exposure. In particular we have abandoned the transverse palmar incision which was the source of many problems. It created a large dissection and potential dead space in the palm when only a longitudinal exposure was necessary and the very area undermined and thus devitalized is already an area of the palm notorious for its poor blood supply. Next this transverse incision left between it and the digital incisions a tunnel which was difficult of access and yet where many significant lesions of Dupuytren's contracture are found and particularly important displacements of the neurovascular bundle can occur. Finally the extension of the fingers tends to pull apart this transverse palmar wound and fear of disruption produced a reluctance to make full postoperative finger movements.

We prefer to use sinuous incisions running from the finger into the palm roughly along the longitudinal axis but obtaining in this way direct exposure of the whole pattern of lesions and their related neurovascular bundles, with limited dissection of skin flaps, healing without undue longitudinal traction and above all a great freedom of application to individual lesions. Thus it permits all types of fasciectomy within the finger and within the palm. Such digitopalmar incisions and selective fasciectomies have produced a significant lowering of postoperative complications and skin necrosis and dehiscence in the palm have not been observed and the risk of haematoma has been greatly diminished. Digital skin problems on the other hand have remained, as they tend to arise from the use of Z-plasties so that we are making more and more use of free skin grafts in the finger, particularly when the skin is infiltrated and unsuitable for the formation of flaps.

Skin closure has concerned surgeons for a long time particularly in regard to excision and conservation of the skin. Some follow the example of Berger (1892) and Lexer (1831) in freely using skin excision because preserving abnormal skin leads to problems in healing, limitation of movement and scar contractures along with the risk of recurrence. Others however, carefully conserve all involved skin and introduce methods of local rearrangement rather than use free grafts which they regard as not only unnecessary but actually dangerous because they feel this invites complications from the poor quality of the graft bed, the inferior skin introduced and the prolonged postoperative period of immobilization.

It is often claimed that excision of the skin on grounds of dermal involvement amounts to an unnecessary sacrifice because the involved skin will return in a large degree to its previous normal elasticity. This is, however, not always true, particularly when the flexion deformity has been severe, and simple closure of a transverse palmar wound means keeping the fingers flexed to lessen the longitudinal tension and introduces the possibility of permanent postoperative stiffness. The introduction of additional skin as grafts appears amply justified in certain cases. However, McCash after palmar fasciectomy and correction of M.P. deformity makes no effort at skin closure and awaits second intention healing of the palmar wound while holding the fingers extended in a night splint to prevent recurrence of the deformity. Certainly the major complications of skin closure, namely haematoma and skin necrosis are avoided by his lack of skin closure in the palm.

In addition to the value of adding free skin grafts seems to introduce a novel and important attribute. Several authors (Piulachs and Mir y Mir, Gordon, and Hueston) have observed that recurrences do not occur in those areas where free grafts have been introduced whereas the adjacent retained areas have become invaded.

These observations have led Hueston to recommend the replacement of infiltrated skin by free skin grafts in most cases where recurrences have occurred already, or even during a primary procedure when, in a young patient, he believes there exists a sufficiently severe Dupuytren's diathesis to make an early postoperative recurrence seem likely.

Gonzalez uses free grafts in the treatment of Dupuytren's contracture in much the same way as one would use them in the correction of burn scar contractures of the finger, by dividing transversely across a band at the point of maximum tension and inserting a full thickness free graft.

All these points have been more extensively discussed by their authors in other chapters of this monograph but they are obviously of great importance not only from the point of view of aetiology but also in considering our surgical management.

DISCUSSION

It would appear that the confrontation between extensive and limited fasciectomies has been exaggerated in its significance and the argument advanced by one or other side is often too partisan.

The operative complications of extensive fasciectomy are to an overwhelming degree more due to the use of a transverse palmar incision than to the extent of the fasciectomy. Nevertheless it appears both logical and reasonable to admit that postoperative complications are less common, and return to work more rapid after the more limited operation even though they are followed by higher incidence of postoperative extension of the disease.

An excessive attention appears to have been directed towards the treatment of the purely fascial lesions and, while these two opposing schools of thought in regard to the amount of palmar fascia to be excised differ in that single regard, they reinforce one another in every other regard, particularly when asserting the indica-

tions for application of surgery to any particular case.

Dupuytren's contracture is not confined purely to fascial lesions, and other factors also play an important role in establishing the prognosis—some general factors are as yet poorly understood and impossible to treat therapeutically but the state of the skin and subcutaneous tissue is on the contrary easy to assess, but appears to be often inadequately appreciated. In fact most of the complications attributed to the extent of the fasciectomy could be due to poor selection and consideration of these other factors at the time of operation.

It is just as wrong to recommend extensive fasciectomy under the pretext of providing prophylaxis as it is to recommend a limited fasciectomy, accepting a higher proportion of recurrences, on the basis of simplicity and postoperative safety. It is necessary to take into account that dissection for recurrences as a secondary procedure is often extremely tedious, recurrent tissues are intimately involving ligaments, nerves and flexor sheaths and thus the treatment of Dupuytren's contracture must be selective from all points of view so that the right operation is selected for every particular patient. There is no place for a routine operation. The selective surgery must consider the patient's age, the aetiological factors, the extent of the lesions and their distribution and the condition of the skin and joints.

At the risk of appearing too rigid it is possible to summarize the indications for operations:

1. No operative treatment is carried out in the presence of palmar nodules without deformity of the fingers or loss of function of the hand.

2. Surgery is avoided whenever possible in the presence of trophic and vasomotor disorders of the hand which are manifested by coolness, cyanosis and oedema. Advanced age and some associated conditions such as epilepsy and chronic alcoholism also constitute unfavourable prognostic factors as described by Hueston elsewhere in this volume. These, however, must be weighted against the progress of the disease and the functional loss so that severe deformities in some cases may be of little inconvenience to the patient and can be left unoperated whereas in other patients rapid progress towards uncorrectable joint deformity in several fingers may lead others to require limited surgery in the presence of obviously unfavourable prognostic factors.

3. Palmar fasciotomies followed by extension of the fingers in a traction splint are reserved for (a) cases where one would prefer to have avoided operation at all but the local conditions demand it. It is particularly suitable for cases with retraction of the M.P. joints and prominent palmar bands which are well defined; it has very little action on the interphalangeal joints, but of course can be associated if necessary with digital fasciectomy; (b) cases where fasciectomy should suffice on its own

or as a preliminary to a more extensive later fasciectomy where the flexion deformity of the fingers has produced such maceration of the skin that the digital dissections have to be postponed for a few weeks after the preliminary opening up of the fingers obtained by the fasciotomy; (c) fasciotomies are contraindicated in the fingers because of the danger of dividing the digital nerves.

4. Fasciectomies are carried out in other cases and rather than 'partial and total' fasciectomies, we prefer to refer to 'limited or extensive' operations.

We use an extensive operation, including all the detectable palmar lesions and extending the fasciectomy for preference over the three ulnar rays of the palmar space as well as the hypothenar fascia and all involved fingers, whenever the operative conditions permit—that is in healthy patients relatively young, with supple skin. If the skin is infiltrated and the disease has started unusually early under 40 years of age, and particularly if other signs of Dupuytren's diathesis lead one to fear recurrences we would, like Hueston, consider excision of the overlying skin and a free graft replacement Excision of the skin, however, is not often carried out except in cases of recurrence.

Limited operations involves only an excision of the aponeurosis in the region of the obvious clinical lesions and is indicated (a) whenever one fears a local complication and particularly therefore when the skin is poorly vascularized, thick and adherent to the underlying lesion and (b) when the general conditions contraindicate the more extensive lesions, such as advanced age or concomitant disease and (c) when the local conditions contraindicate an extensive palmar fasciectomy such as diffuse lesions in the palm or extensive contractions of the interphalangeal joints.

5. Arthrotomies, arthrodeses and amputation. When the digital flexion deformity is severe and particularly when it is mainly at the P.I.P. joints it is necessary to warn the patient beforehand that correction of these deformities may be incomplete after simple fasciectomy and it should be discussed with him before the operation that there are other possibilities for more permanent correction of the deformity (a) frequently after careful digital fasciectomy and if necessary excision of the fibrous flexor sheath, it is possible to obtain full extension of the finger despite a very severe preoperative flexion deformity; but there will remain a tendency

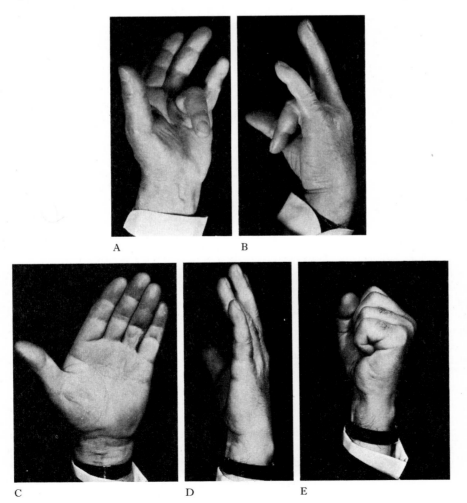

A   B

C   D   E

Figure 12.1
Dupuytren's disease in a man of 55 years with severe contracture of the ring finger. Pre-operative formula O, O, O, 4PD+, IP = 5; i.e. no lesion on the thumb, index and middle finger; 70° deformity of the metacarpophalangeal joint of the ring finger and 90° at its proximal interphalangeal joint giving a total of 160° of retration which = stage 4. The + sign indicates the predominance of the lesion on the proximal interphalangeal level and the total 5 represents the addition of deformities of both ring (4) and little (1) fingers.

This patient has been operated on by digitopalmar approach with limited fasciectomy in the palm extending into the base of the ring finger. Despite fasciectomy about 40° PIP flexion deformity remains and was not correctable by resection of the fibrous flexor sheath over the proximal phalanx. A Kirschner wire had to be inserted obliquely across the interphalangeal joint to combat the tendency for the flexor tendons to reproduce the deformity. This was left for 1 week and helped the healing of the Z-plasty in the skin. Post-operative formula O, O, O, ID, O = 1; gain from the operation is clearly 5 − 1 = 4. This postoperative formula if there persists no limitation of flexion post-operatively. Such a limitation of flexion would be represented by the letter L.

for this finger to return spontaneously to its previous flexion because of flexor muscle contracture and it is necessary to combat this strenuously by early application of elastic traction splints to retain extension postoperatively. Postoperative immobilization of the P.I.P. joint for one week and postoperatively by Kirschner wire placed obliquely, can be useful here and the risk of producing stiffness by this manoeuvre is slight if the joint has not been opened and if healing is early and uneventful: (b) when it has been necessary to open a joint for one week and postoperatively by a Kirschner operative stiffness in extension is much greater and it is better that the patient should be warned about this preoperatively. It should be emphasized to the patient that from the functional point of view it is better to have a loss of extension of the fingers than a loss of flexion: (c) finally it may be necessary to discuss those procedures which produce permanent correction of the flexion deformity, although at the same time producing permanent functional loss from eliminating flexion— namely arthrodesis of the P.I.P. joint or amputation. These more mutilating procedures are not often considered except in cases of recurrence.

CONCLUSIONS

The principles guiding the surgical treatment of Dupuytren's contracture aim in the first place to produce the best functional result and in the second place to prevent recurrences.

They aim to offer the patient the most complete correction that the state of the patient will allow and this assessment can be extremely delicate. Each operation must be chosen and adapted to allow the maximum improvement without complications.

REFERENCES

GORDON, S. (1957). Dupuytren's contracture: recurrence and extension following surgical treatment. *British Journal of Plastic Surgery, 9*, 286.

GOSSET, J. (1973). Dupuytren's disease and anatomy of the palmodigital aponeuroses. This volume.

HAKSTIAN, R. W. (1967). Late results of extensive fasciectomy. In *Maladie de Dupuytren*, 1st edn. Groupe d'Etude de la Main. Paris: Expansion Scientific Française.

HUESTON, J. T. (1962). Digital Wolfe grafts in recurrent Dupuytren's contracture. *Plastic and Reconstructive Surgery, 29*, 342.

HUESTON, J. T. (1963). *Dupuytren's Contracture*. Edinburgh: Livingstone.

HUESTON, J. T. (1967). Prognosis as a guide to the timing and extent of surgery in Dupuytren's contracture. In *Maladie de Dupuytren*, 1st edn., p. 69. Groupe d'Etude de la Main. Paris: Expansion Scientific Française.

LEXER, E. (1931). *Die gesamte Wiederherstillungschirurgie*, 2nd edn., vol. 2. Leipzig:

MILLESI, H. (1973). The clinical and morphological course of Dupuytren's disease. This volume.

NEZELOF, C. (1973). Histological aspects of Dupuytren's contracture. This volume.

PIULACHS, P. & MIR y MIR, L. (1952). Consideraciones sobre la enfermedad de Dupuytren. *Folia clinica internacional (Barcelona), 2*, 8.

SHAW, M. & EASTWOOD, D. (1952). Dupuytren's contracture. A selective approach to treatment. *British Journal of Plastic Surgery, 28*, 2.

SKOOG, T. (1973). Dupuytren's contracture: pathogenesis and surgical treatment. This volume.

THOMINE, J. M. (1964). Contribution à l'étude de la maladie de Dupuytren et son traitement chirurgical. Thesis, Paris.

THOMINE, J. M. (1965). Conjonctifs d'envelopes des doigts et squelette fibreux des commissures interdigital. *Annales de Chirurgie plastique, 10* (3), 194.

TUBIANA, R. (1963). Les temps cutanés dans le traitment chirurgical de la maladie de Dupuytren. *Annales de Chirurgie plastique, 8* (3), 157–168.

TUBIANA, R. (1964a). Le traitement sélectif de la maladie de Dupuytren. *Revue de Chirurgie orthopedique et reparatrice de l'Appareil moteur, 50* (3), 311–334.

TUBIANA, R. (1964b). Limited and extensive operations in Dupuytren's contracture. *Surgical Clinics of North America, 44*, 1072–1080.

TUBIANA, R., THOMINE, J. M. & BROWN, S. (1967). Complications in surgery of Dupuytren's contracture. *Plastic and Reconstructive Surgery, 39* (6), 603–612.

13. LATE RESULTS OF EXTENSIVE FASCIECTOMY

R. W. Hakstian

Just as the progress of untreated Dupuytren's disease still remains unpredictable so there exists uncertainty and insufficient knowledge concerning its evolution following surgery. Although surgical intervention is generally accepted as an essential modality in the successful management of the condition, the significance of the surgical episode in the course of the disease is not well known. How does surgery alter the evolution of the lesions in the individual case? Can it have a curative effect or does it simply retard the development of functionally disabling contracture? Is it possible that surgery may aggravate the disease and cause a more rapid development of deformity than would have occurred had it not been performed?

Most case reviews which attempt to assess the results of surgery fail to provide an evaluation far enough removed from the operation. These short term reviews indicate that redevelopment of disease following both limited and extensive fasciectomy is of minor proportions. It is, however, rather alarming to study the excellent long term reviews of Hueston which suggest that a very low percentage of hands remain free of disease following fasciectomy. While the effectiveness of the limited and radical procedures is difficult to compare in these series, because of the difference of indications, there was a high frequency of renewed disease following both. The long term follow-up of partial fasciectomy cases indicated that disease redeveloped in 80 per cent of hands.

An unique opportunity existed for a long term review by an impartial observer when the records of those patients operated on by Sir Archibald McIndoe at the Queen Victoria Hospital, England, were available to the author. The following review material consists of the results of surgery of 51 patients (87 hands). The time of review was from 5 to 25 years after initial surgery, (Mean 11·1 years). Those patients who were examined did not constitute a purely random sample as certain criteria were imposed in order to reduce the number of variables affecting the evaluation of the surgical procedure. In the first place only those patients having had both palmar and digital involvement were recalled. These hands were operated on by the extensive fasciectomy technique employing a transverse palmar exposure combined with volar digital Z-plasty technique of the involved fingers as described by McIndoe and Beare (1958). In addition all operations, both initial and subsequent were performed by the same surgeon. By selecting the cases for review in this manner it was possible to obtain a fairly homogenous sample and therefore make a better correlation between the operation performed and the results obtained. For each patient the review included an interview, clinical examination of the hands, photography and radiography.

RESULTS OF THE REVIEW

Of the 51 patients seen, 46 were men and 5, women. A family history was present in 14 instances (28 per cent), the mean age of onset was 43·0 years; of operation 48·5 years. Bilateral disease was present in 70·6 per cent of the patients at the time of initial surgery so that 87 hands were involved. Ultimately some hands that had been free of disease became involved so that bilateral Dupuytren's occurred in 84·3 per cent of patients. The study group concerns 73 operated hands.

Not all hands were in the same state of contraction preoperatively. According to the McIndoe and Beare staging, 15 of the operated hands were in stage I; 34, in stage II; 14, in stage III; and 10, in stage IV. In ten of the advanced cases, in addition to the fasciectomy, an amputation of the little finger was performed.

Postoperative care followed a carefully established pattern in all instances. Wound healing was delayed in 1/3 of cases but in only two were the complications of a serious magnitude.

Early recovery of hand function was recorded in the patient's file and was considered normal if all the fingers could be actively flexed into the palm within 6–10 weeks after surgery. By stages there was normal recovery in 87 per cent, 88 percent, 57 per cent and 40 per cent respectively. The functional results following fasciectomy were considered 'excellent' if full flexion and extension of the involved fingers could be achieved with normal power. A 'good' result showed some slight extension or finger spread limitation or incomplete flexion of the involved finger. A 'fair' result indicated partial correction of the deformity together with a flexion deficit or joint stiffness. A result was considered 'poor' if the situation was no improvement on the preoperative disability. The functional results during the first year post operation and at the time of late review

TABLE I   Postoperative course following extensive fasciectomy

	All cases Hands	%
Hands operated upon	73	100
Wound complications	24	34
Results 1 year post O.P.:		
—Excellent	50	69
—Good	20	27
—Fair	3	4
—Poor	0	0
Long-term results 11.1 years:		
—Excellent	36	49
—Good	24	33
—Fair	11	15
—Poor	2	3
Renewed disease:	37	51
—Recurrence	25	34
—Extension	24	33
Clear of disease	36	49
Requiring secondary surgery	18	25
Requiring tertiary surgery	6	8

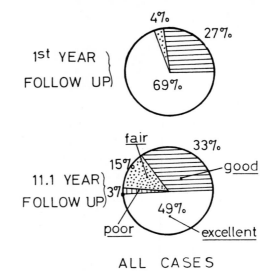

Figure 13.1
Functional results after extensive fasciectomy: Overall result.

are shown in Table 1 and Figs. 1 and 2. (Five hands were reviewed 20–25 years after initial operation; 15, 15–20 years; 25, 10–14 years; 28, 5–9 years). It can be seen that the functional results deteriorated little over the years. There were between 10 and 20 per cent fewer cases in the excellent and good categories at long term follow-up than there had been at first year review. While we are not primarily interested in the subjective results it was extremely interesting to note that very few patients considered their hands normal after operation. The patients often stated that they had given up golf or did less motoring than before the operation and while the reasons tended to be psychological in many instances there were some patients who did complain of tenderness in the palm and loss of suppleness. Good long term results do not reflect the true value of the initial operative

procedure as in 25 per cent of all cases, secondary surgery was necessary and in another 8 per cent, a third operation was required to correct deformity and dysfunction due to renewed disease. Redevelopment of disease was evident in 51 per cent of hands with some showing recurrences, some, extensions and some, both (Tables 1, 2; Fig. 13.3). Generally these occurred within 2 years of initial surgery but in 6 hands (of the 73) there were clinical manifestations of new disease only after 5 years. Therefore 49 per cent of hands were free of disease when examined no sooner than 5 years and as late as 25 years after initial surgery.

The tendency to bilateral involvement, noted by others, was confirmed in this study. Renewed disease almost always developed in both hands in the bilaterally operated cases. Of the 72 hands (36 patients with

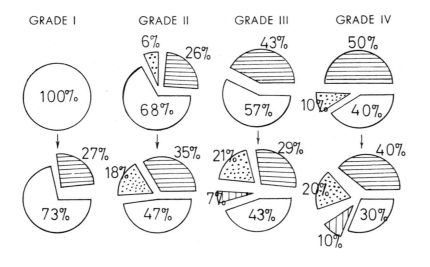

Figure 13.2
Functional result considered according to grade of deformity. Above: One year after operation. Below: 11·1 years (average) after operation. (White = excellent; horizontal hatching = good; dotted = fair; vertical hatching = bad result.)

TABLE 2   The results of extensive fasciectomy

Unilateral involvement			Bilateral involvement	
Hands	%		Hands	%
15	100	Number of hands operated	58	100
6	40	Hands with renewed disease	31	53
3	20	Recurrences	22	38
4	27	Extensions	20	35
9	60	Hands clear of disease	27	47
3	20	Secondary surgery	15	26
0	0	Tertiary surgery	6	10

bilateral disease) 26 (36 per cent remained free of disease with or without operation. When only the operated hands (58) are considered, one finds that 47 per cent remained free of disease. It seems evident that some prophylactic value may be accorded to this operative method.

In the group of 15 patients initially presenting with unilateral disease there were 17 hands that remained free of disease at long term follow-up. These included 8 hands that were never involved with disease at the clinical level and 9 operated hands. The incidence of renewed disease following operation is shown in Table 1.

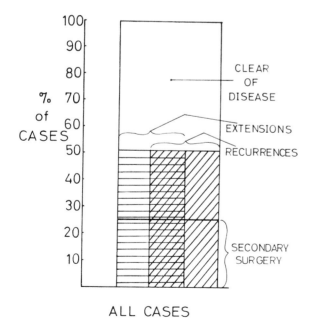

RENEWED DEVELOPMENT OF DISEASE

Figure 13.3
Recurrences—total series

DISCUSSION

(A). PATHOGENESIS OF DUPUYTREN'S DISEASE

While a detailed review of the etiology and evolution of palmar fibromatosis is not in order here, some allusion to recent investigations of others is necessary for the proper evaluation of the results of the present review.

There is general agreement that the disease is a familial one. It is proposed by many that a genetic factor of low penetrance expresses itself in adult life as a fascial susceptibility to some causal agent or other. (There are other inherited diseases which become clinically evident only in adult life such as hereditary hemorrhagic telangiectasia.) The nature of this latter event is not known but there is evidence that it may take the form of mechanical stress (repeated minor trauma) or of an auto-immune reaction to abnormal collagen.

The microanatomical studies of recent years confirm the presence of at least two histological forms within the diseased tissue. Highly cellular microscopic whorls are seen in early and recurrent disease while elongated lamellar and relatively accelular collagen formations typify long standing lesions. The two forms may be present in the same microscopic field although the latter type is more often seen at the exterior of the specimen. Millesi has pointed to the presence, in specimens studied under the electron microscope, of degenerative collagen forms which he feels may represent the initiating antigenic factor.

Unfortunately there is nothing about the microscopic appearance of this disease in its established form to distinguish it from scar tissue. It seems reasonable to assume therefore that Dupuytren's disease represents a derangement of collagen formation. There is excessive connective tissue synthesis in response to some stimulus or other as yet undetermined. The situation resembles that of hypertrophic scarring and keloid formation and of excessive adhesion formation following tendon or joint trauma either accidental or surgical. Certainly in these conditions, repeated intervention is associated with an even greater accumulation of connective tissue.

(B). EXTENT OF FASCIECTOMY

The controversy over the relative merits of partial and radical fasciectomy which developed in the 1950's has served some useful purposes. It has led to a clarification of the clinical indications for the various procedures as it became evident that too many variables existed to permit routine application of any one operation. The need was also made obvious for more careful study of the normal anatomy of the palmar aponeurosis as well as of the diseased tissue and sources of renewed disease.

Recent careful studies have shown that the palmar aponeurosis is a complex tissue with many superficial and deep attachments, both proximally and distally.

Renewed disease may develop from both aponeurotic and subcutaneous sources.

At the present time the surgical treatment of Dupuytren's contracture represents a compromise. Fasciectomy limited to the immediately diseased area corrects the clinical manifestation of the disease but is followed by a high incidence of renewed disease requiring subsequent surgery. Since the scarring effect of this is additive, a serious progression of the disease is likely. On the other hand some prophylactic value is attributed to extensive fasciectomy and our results support this contention. However, such wide dissection, which never represents total removal, of course, may be associated with wound healing complications that leave as their mark excessive scar tissue. This scar may not represent renewed Dupuytren's disease but it certainly serves the same role in re-establishing disability in the hand.

Examination of the knowledge we now possess indicates that an entirely satisfactory solution of the problem does not exist. However, consideration of the known facts does permit the formation of a guide management:

1. Multiple operations lead to successively poorer results.
2. Some prophylactic value can be attributed to extensive surgical resection.
3. Wound healing complications increase as the extent of the dissection increases and devaluate the operative result.
4. Under the best of circumstances, half the hands operated on once will redevelop disease and two thirds of these will require more surgery to correct functional disability.

With an expected control rate of less than 50 per cent under favourable conditions one must question the therapeutic modality. Indeed it does seem that we can not count on surgical resection for a definitive cure in this disease. After all it is not technically possible to remove all the potential sources of recurrence or extension. Probably the cure of this condition will be in the nature of a biochemical modality designed to modify collagen formation. At that time surgery may still have a place in removing the diseased tissue immediately responsible for the deformity. In the meantime we must do the best we can, as in the surgery of neoplasms, with our operative techniques. It appears evident that with all factors being equal (re: age, general condition, associated diseases, etc.) the best chance for success exists with a single extensive fasciectomy performed skilfully and with great attention to postoperative care, accompanied by early mobilization and followed in later years with limited resections of disability caused by scar tissue or renewed disease.

SUMMARY

A long term review has been made of 87 hand operations performed for Dupuytren's disease. In all cases an extensive fasciectomy was performed by the same surgeon. The duration between initial operation and follow-up was between 5 and 25 years and averaged 11·1 years.

It was found that 49 per cent of hands were free of disease at the clinical level following this intervention.

Renewed disease in the form of recurrences or extensions developed in 51 per cent of hands. Secondary and tertiary surgery was necessary in two thirds of these cases to further check the progress of the disease and insure useful hand function.

Allusion is made to the long-term reviews of Hueston. Comparison with the statistics for redevelopment of disease following limited fasciectomy is the basis for the conclusion that extensive fasciectomy does have more prophylactic value than limited fasciectomy.

CONCLUSION

Surgery alone can not be expected to produce routine cures in Dupuytren's disease.

The evolution of the disease can be modified by operation in many cases and more normal hand function restored. Even when this is of a temporary nature it will be more acceptable to the patient than the crippling disability of established Dupuytren's contracture.

Extensive surgical dissection may be complicated by serious wound healing problems that lead to excessive scar tissue formation and early return of deformity and disability in the hand.

REFERENCES

BUNNELL, S. (1956). *Surgery of the Hand,* 3rd edn. Philadelphia: Lippincott.

CLARKSON, P. (1963). *British Journal of Plastic Surgery,* **16,** 273.

CONWAY, H., GILLETTE, R. W., SMITH, J. W. & FINDLEY, A. (1960). *Plastic and Reconstructive Surgery,* **25,** 117.

FREEHAFER, A. A. & STRONG, J. M. (1963). *Journal of Bone and Joint Surgery,* **45A,** 1207.

HAMLIN, E. (1962). *Annals of Surgery,* **155,** 454.

HUESTON, J. T. (1961). *Plastic and Reconstructive Surgery,* **27,** 569.

HUESTON, J. T. (1963). *Plastic and Reconstructive Surgery,* **31,** 66.

HUESTON, J. T. (1964). Royal College of Surgeons: Hunterian Lecture, 8th October.

LARSEN, R. D. & POSCH, J. L. (1958). *Journal of Bone and Joint Surgery,* **40A,** 773.

LARSEN, R. D., TAKAGISHI, N. & POSCH, J. L. (1960). *Journal of Bone and Joint Surgery,* **42A,** 993.

MILLESI, H. (1962). The Second Hand Club, Paris Meeting.

McINDOE, SIR ARCHIBALD H. & BEARE, R. L. B. (1958). *American Journal of Surgery,* **95,** 197.

PALETTA, F. X. (1963). *Transactions of the International Society of Plastic Surgery,* p. 416. Amsterdam: Exerpta Medica.

SHAW, M. H. (1964). *Postgraduate Medical Journal,* **40,** 287.

SKOOG, T. (1943). *Acta chirurgica scandinavica,* **96,** Suppl. 139.

SKOOG, T. (1963). *Plastic and Reconstructive Surgery,* **31,** 258.

TUBIANA, R. (1955). *Journal of Bone and Joint Surgery,* **37A,** 1155.

TUBIANA, R. (1964). *Revue de Chirurgie orthopédique et réparatrice de l'Appareil moteur,* **50,** 311.

WANG, K. H., MACOMBER, W. B., STEIN, A., RAJPAL, R. & HEFFERNAN, A. (1960). *Plastic and Reconstructive Surgery,* **25,** 323.

14. SURGICAL TREATMENT OF DUPUYTREN'S CONTRACTURE: TECHNIQUE OF FASCIOTOMY AND FASCIECTOMY

Raoul Tubiana and Jean-Michel Thomine

The line of treatment which we have adopted in recent years for Dupuytren's contracture is based on a certain conception of the disease and also on repeated reviewing of fasciectomies performed in the past.

As far as the aetiology of the disease is concerned, we know few solid facts capable of influencing treatment; the latter therefore remains primarily symptomatic. Our knowledge of the natural history is still full of gaps. We are not entirely convinced by J. Hueston's theories, which suggest an extra-aponeurotic origin of the disease, and we still believe that the disease process originates within the 'aponeurotic skeleton', and, as a result, that excision of the lesions requires a *systematic dissection of anatomical structures,* especially in the commissures and digital fascia.

As a rule, the extent of a fasciectomy will depend on the risks of recurrence (diathesis), the risks of complications (in the skin in particular) and on the age of the patient. Correction of the deformities rather than prophylaxis remains the primary goal when one decides how wide an excision shall be.

But in view of the frequency and severity of digital recurrences we tend to extend our dissections and widen our excisions at the level of the fingers. Besides, well planned wider excisions at the fingers allow for better correction of deformities. Indeed we have often been surprised by the accepted tendency to perform an extensive and systematic excision of palmar lesions while digital lesions are seldom and only partially dealt with.

On the other hand, considering that primary lesions rarely involve the thumb and index finger, we limit 'extensive resections' to the three ulnar interosseus spaces and their corresponding pretendinous bands unless these two digits are directly affected.

ANAESTHESIA AND POSITIONING OF THE PATIENT

We prefer to operate under general anaesthesia whenever the general condition of the patient will allow it. We are not entirely convinced by the theory of some authors that local or regional anaesthesia may help in preventing postoperative vascular complications. We believe that most of these can be avoided by a thorough preoperative assessment of the trophic state of the hand, by careful surgery, and by adequate postoperative care supervised by the surgeon himself.

The operation takes place under a tourniquet. This can be placed without the use of an Esmarch bandage if the limb is previously held suspended. Dissection and haemostasis are made easier if a small quantity of blood is allowed to remain in the vessels. The cuff is inflated up to a pressure some 5 to 10 mm above the patient's systolic pressure, and in most patients, can be left in place, if necessary, for $1\frac{1}{2}$ hours. If need be, it can be let down and reinflated 10 minutes later.

The patient is placed in the dorsal position, the upper limb resting on a table connected to the operating table. The hand is held down, with the fingers wide apart and in maximum extension, by a malleable splint of our own design which has the advantage over lead splints that it can be used to separate the fingers from one another. The fingers are fixed to it by means of rubber rings cut from operating gloves.

The first stage of the operation consists in *marking out the incision,* taking into account the exposure required and the problems of closure. This must be carefully thought out and not improvised after the tourniquet is already inflated.

When severe retraction is present, the incision cannot be completely marked out until the metacarpophalangeal joint has been partially straightened. Through the initial part of the incision a palmar fasciotomy can be carried out which in turn facilitated the marking out of the digital incision and the rest of the operation.

In some cases, the fasciotomy is but a prelude to a secondary fasciectomy, allowing the treatment of macerated skin which would make immediate excision of lesions a risky procedure.

SURGICAL TECHNIQUES

Fasciotomy. This is a relatively minor procedure reserved for the more prominent and localized bands. We believe that it has a place only in the palm, as in the fingers, the relationships between the neurovascular bundles and the hypertrophic fascial bands are extremely variable.

To be safe, this procedure must be carried out through a skin incision and not blindly. We like to use small longitudinal incisions made along the palmar bands to be divided. Transverse incisions tend to gape during extension and should be avoided.

In less advanced cases, fasciotomy will straighten out the M.P. joints and, less frequently, restore some freedom of movement at the proximal I.P. joint. This gain must be maintained by early elastic bracing. If required, still greater freedom can be achieved by an open excision of the digital aponeurotic lesions.

Fasciectomy. We shall consider in turn the problems of exposure, excision of aponeurotic lesions, ways of dealing with extra-aponeurotic causes of retraction, skin coverage following digital extension, hemostasis, and postoperative care.

(A) EXPOSURE OF LESIONS

We always use *digitopalmar incisions,* which allow whole-length dissection of the lesions and good exposure of the neurovascular bundles throughout their course. Blind dissection at the base of the most severely affected finger, as occurs with transverse palmar incisions, is thus avoided. The palmar incision, the overall direction of which is longitudinal, is continued along the most severely affected finger. Separate incisions can be used, for the other fingers, as necessary.

MARKING OUT THE PALMAR INCISION

Sinuous longitudinal incisions run along the flexion creases for part of their course. In particular the proximal portion often follows the hypothenar crease. The wider the proposed fasciectomy, the more sinuous the incision. It is worth emphasizing here that these incisions permit as extensive a palmar resection as a transverse incision.

When marking out the exposure one should avoid placing the bow string of the incision alongside a band adherent to the skin, as dissection close to the skin interferes with the blood supply. It is preferable to get the incision to coincide with the linear adhesions, and, if required, to excise the devitalized edges of the wound.

In an attempt to preserve the blood supply to the skin, it is worth trying to spare some of the perforating vessels which run through the aponeurosis to the teguments.

The palmar incision ends by joining the proximal flexor crease of the finger which it follows for a short distance before becoming continuous with the digital incision.

A single digitopalmar incision is usually sufficient, although when required, a double one may be used as long as the intervening bridge of skin is not too narrow. The second incision may be shorter as it only serves to give access to the more distal palmar lesions. Thus an incision on the ulnar border of the little finger may be continued into the hypothenar region when the main incision is directed towards another finger.

Lesions of the thumb, index finger and adjacent palmar areas must be dealt with through separate incisions.

The fibrous band causing flexion of the thumb often runs into the thenar eminence and can be approached through a digitopalmar incision which crosses the digitopalmar flexion crease. The band of the 1st web space frequently runs along the lateral aspect of the index; it is exposed through an incision made along the crest of the commissure, continued on the lateral aspect of the finger, and closed by Z-plasty.

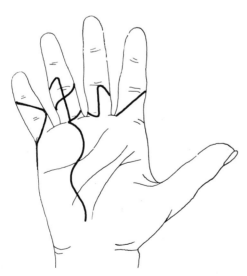

Figure 14.1
The typical outline of the digitopalmar exposure is outlined on the ring finger and would be closed with double Z-plasty. The adjacent fingers show variations of exposure either isolated of in continuity with a palmar incision.

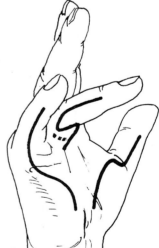

Figure 14.2
A digitopalmar incision is shown on the little finger; the lateral digital exposure is extended across the palmar aspect of the hypothenar eminence. A Z-incision is shown on the proximal segment of the ring finger and can be extended onto the middle segment from its lateral end. On the thumb an S incision allowing exposure of a band on the lateral aspect of the thumb into the palm.

Digital incisions. Each incision has its own advantages.

1. *A midline incision,* continued if required over the middle phalanx, gives equal access to both sides of the finger, but, to avoid retraction, it must be closed by one or more Z-plasties. Exposure is further improved if the flaps of the Z are raised at the beginning of the operation.

However, small flaps composed from skin with mediocre vascularity can present problems of wound healing. Such problems should be foreseen and other methods of wound closure used.

2. *A lateral incision* on the dorsopalmar line does not give rise to cicatricial retraction. It provides adequate exposure if preoperative retraction is not too severe, and if it is made on the more affected side. A Z-plasty may be added, but the gain in length is less than after a midline incision.

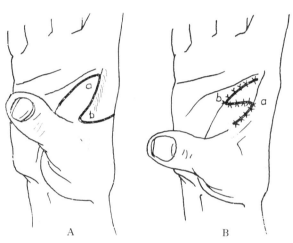

Figure 14.3
Exposure of bands in the first web space; a Z-plasty is employed with flaps outlined as in A; and B, allowing extension if necessary onto the base of the index.

3. *Diagonal incision.* This crosses the palmar aspect of the phalanx obliquely from one flexion crease to the next. If used in continuity with a palmar incision, it gives a good exposure of the proximal phalanx and healing is usually good. It may be continued over the middle phalanx either in a reverse oblique direction or as a lateral incision. Exposure at the base of the resulting flap is excellent and good access is provided on the lateral aspect of the finger.

FASCIAL EXCISION

Excision follows the structural anatomy; its extent will depend on the clinical findings, on knowledge of the mechanism of each deformity, and lastly on prophylactic considerations. Three areas of excision may be distinguished: the palm, the commissural zones including the base of the finger, and the finger proper. During a

dissection, great care must be taken to preserve the nerves and arteries, and to spare the gliding apparatus of the tendons.

(A) THE PALM

The proximal limit of a fasciectomy. Recurrences and extensions are so infrequent in the most proximal part of the palm that resection at the apex of the aponeurotic triangle is seldom indicated.

There is little point therefore in going beyond the line of the abducted thumb (i.e. just above the superficial palmar arch), except in the rare cases of carpal tunnel or canal of Guyon compression symptoms, in which the incision should be extended just above the wrist.

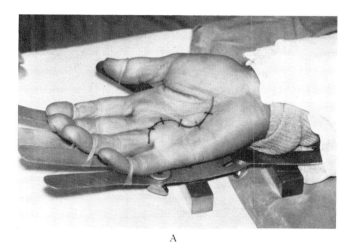

A

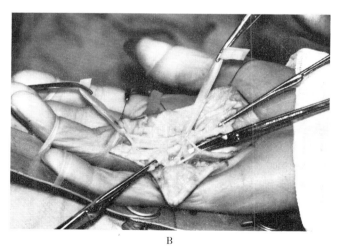

B

Figure 14.4
A. The sinuous digitopalmar incision is outlined. Digital lesion will be exposed by a short angled distal extension.
B. The exposure obtained through this incision. Note the dissection in the 4th web space where the fasciectomy is in progress. The skin flaps are retracted with sutures and the neurovascular pedicles by rubber bands.

The distal limit of a fasciectomy. Palmar fasciectomy is continued into the finger whenever required, the retraction bands being dissected in continuity. The middle palmar aponeurosis, the digital fascia of the most affected finger and the fibrous tissue of the adjacent commissures are thus excised in one piece ('en bloc'). In the other fingers, the dissection stops at the interdigital palmar ligament and only involves the pretendinous bands; the transverse palmar ligament is not systematically preserved, as Skoog suggests.

The width of the fasciectomy. This varies according to the surgeon's ideas about prophylaxis. In a 'radical' resection, we include the middle palmar aponeurosis but not the pretendinous band of the index. Otherwise we only excise a strip of healthy aponeurosis around the pathological structures.

The depth of the fasciectomy. The resection must include the paratendinous septa and the walls of the lumbrical and neurovascular tunnels which are usually continuous with the fibrous structures of the fingers. It extends down to, but does not include, the deep aponeurosis which is preserved. Excision of these palmar structures will usually correct M.P. deformities, and, in certain cases, produce some degree of extension in the proximal I.P. joint. The retractions are caused on the one hand by the presence of palmar bands and on the other by involvement of the sagittal septa. But flexion of the proximal I.P. joints is produced also by direct involvement of the digital and commissural fascia.

(B) THE WEB SPACES AND BASES OF THE FINGERS

This region must be exposed and explored even if no limitation of abduction has been detected clinically in the interdigital web.

An important fascial confluence lies in the commissure (described elsewhere in this monograph). At this point, where the collateral bundles may undergo pathological deviations, three aponeurotic structures converge: through these the fibrous apparatus of the palm mingles with the digital fascia and becomes inserted on the skeleton. The first one is sagittal and continues the paratendinous fibrous septum distally. Normally quite thin in the healthy hand and only reinforced by a few longitudinal fibres from the bands of the palmar aponeurosis, it is frequently the site of retraction in Dupuytren's contracture. In the digital fascia, it is continued deep to the neurovascular bundle.

The second structure, which is frontal, is the continuation at the commissure of the deep palmar aponeurosis. The third connective tissue sheet is anterolateral; it is the palmar interdigital or natatory ligament which closes the commissure anteriorly and crosses over the tendons. A large number of its fibres run into the digital fascia along the lateral and posterior aspects of the neurovascular bundles whose sheaths they reinforce. Through the digital fascia which is tethered on its deep surface to the lateral border of the proximal phalanx, retraction of these structures can flex the finger. This is why division of the pretendinous bands and even of the paratendinous septa may not free the M.P. joints if the fibrous tissue of the commissure, tethered to the palm, is not excised.

We regard the dissection of the web spaces on either side of the retracted finger as an important step. This involves subcutaneous undermining, which despite the absence of a intervening fatty layer, is quite easily performed.

We must stress the fact that it is only at the level of the base of the finger that the collateral bundles become intimately connected with the pathological structures while, in the palm, they are quite separate. It is also worth noting that the artery and the nerve do not divide at the same level. The artery often bifurcates late, at a

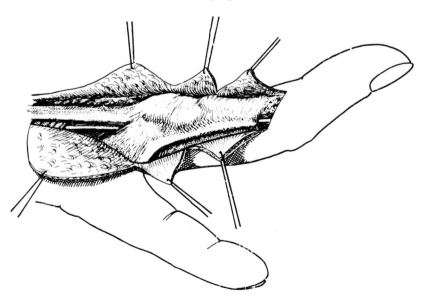

Figure 14.5
Diagram of a fasciectomy in continuity. The Z-flaps in the finger have been raised at the beginning of the exposure and give excellent access to the digital lesions and those in the web space.

wide angle, and is therefore exposed to accidental division when surgical attention is concentrated on the nerve (especially as hypertrophic fibrous tissue is often interposed between the separate bifurcations of artery and nerve).

For these reasons we regard as imperative a direct approach which is only possible through a digito-palmar incision.

(C) EXCISION IN THE DIGITS

This begins with the commissural stage described above. Anatomical studies show that for the proximal phalanx at least, the resection can be preplanned as accurately as for the other operative stages. It must include the aponeurotic 'wallet' formed, on the palmar aspect of the finger, by the two neurovascular sheaths and the middle sheet connecting them. Such a resection is essential in most interphalangeal deformities produced by retraction of digital fascia. The latter often becomes stuck on to the anterior aspect of the tendon sheath, just beyond the proximal I.P. joint. At this point, under normal anatomical conditions, the digital fascia adheres to the fibrous flexor sheath, while elsewhere

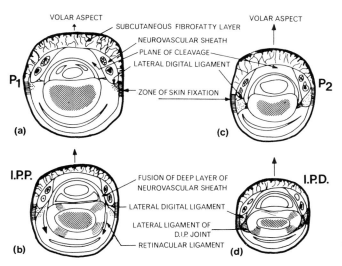

Figure 14.6
Transverse sections at different levels of the finger.

these structures are separated by a cleavable plane usually unaffected by the disease. Dissection of nodules and digital bands usually leads to this level where the collateral nerves and arteries are most at risk. They may be pulled towards the midline by retraction of their digital fascial covering, and as they emerge unexpectedly from their protective fascia they become exposed to inadvertent damage even when the skin incision is made. Hence the importance of identifying arteries and nerves in healthy areas and using loops of rubber as markers.

(D) AT THE LEVEL OF THE 5th FINGER

In addition to the corresponding fibrous structures in the other fingers, there is here a medial band which is almost constant, stretching between the digital fascia of the proximal phalanx and the hypothenar apon-eurosis, it lies superficial to the medial neurovascular bundle, closely adherent to the tendon of abductor digiti minimi. This structure, which is sometimes quite thick, keeps the M.P. joint of the 5th finger flexed, and if the fourth interdigital web is not invaded by fibrosis, it may pull the 5th finger into abduction. In the more advanced cases, it is in the 5th finger that hyperextension of the distal I.P. joint is most frequently encountered.

The mechanism of hyperextension of the distal I.P. joint in Dupuytren's contracture is poorly understood. We believe that there is at least one anatomical explanation. At the level of the proximal I.P. joint the digital fascia is closely related to the retinacular ligament of Landsmeer. This relationship is achieved via the retro-vascular fibrous reinforcement which we call 'digital retrovascular fibrous band'. This band includes a bundle which belongs to the proximal phalanx and crosses the ligament of Landsmeer superficially, becoming adherent to this ligament over several milli-metres. Beyond the ligament, the fibrous band mingles with the fibrous bundle belonging to the middle phalanx. It is conceivable therefore that a retracted digital fascia, thus fixed to the retinacular ligament, might put its oblique fibres on the stretch with resulting hyper-extension of the distal I.P. joint. This hypothesis seems more plausible than direct involvement of the ligament, which flexion of the proximal I.P. joint would rather tend to relax. It seems to us therefore that hyper-extension should be corrected by freeing the oblique retinacular ligament. This requires extensive dissection towards the dorsal aspect of the finger. Because of joint stiffness, however, excising the fibrous bands does not necessarily restore joint mobility; the extension deform-ity is less crippling than the opposite deformity.

(E) AT THE LEVEL OF THE THUMB

Retractions involving the thumb are far from rare and are of two types:

1. Flexion of the metacarpophalangeal joint, with or without flexion of the I.P. joint, due to a longitudinal anterolateral band running from the thenar aponeurosis to the lateral aspects of the phalanges. Its resection requires an incision which crosses the proximal flexion crease of the thumb 'en bayonet'. Only the pathological tissues need be excised.

2. The commissural band consists of a small antero-medial fibrous band which is sometimes continuous with a band on the anterolateral aspect of the index. This band is troublesome as it prevents separation of the thumb from the palm. A wide approach, using a Z-

incision, is usually required. The transverse arm of the Z follows the crest of the commissure: raising of the flaps gives adequate exposure, and by closing them in Z a skin gain will be achieved at the first commissure.

EXTRA-APONEUROTIC RETRACTIONS

Excision of fibrous structures directly involved in the disease process is not itself sufficient to correct all deformities especially in advanced cases, as there exist extra-aponeurotic causes for finger deformities. In practice this is more true of the proximal I.P. joint as the anatomical architecture of the M.P. joint is such that its collateral ligaments are kept at maximal length during flexion.

These permanent flexion deformities of the proximal I.P. joint are related to two factors: retraction of the fibrous flexor sheath and of the capsuloligamentous apparatus.

Retraction of the fibrous flexor sheath must be dealt with first. During excision of the aponeurosis, a portion of

the adherent sheath is sometimes removed with the fascia, leaving a hole which gapes during extension of the finger. The first step consists in incising the sheath transversely at the level of the I.P. joint and if this proves insufficient, a partial excision is performed.

When it is clear that the fibrous flexor sheath is not responsible, attention must be turned to the proximal I.P. joint itself. To reduce the risks of postoperative stiffness and to preserve the elements of lateral and anteroposterior stability of the joint, the 'arthrolysis' must, as much as possible, remain extra-articular. One must start therefore by dividing the accessory phalango-glenoid ligaments, and then free the glenoid fibro-cartilage proximally. Division of the collateral ligaments and excision of the volar plate may lead to stiffness and instability.

It must be stressed again that after the more severe retractions have been corrected, the finger may show a tendency to close spontaneously under the action of retracted muscles. Elastic extension braces must then be used to prevent a recurrence of the deformity. In

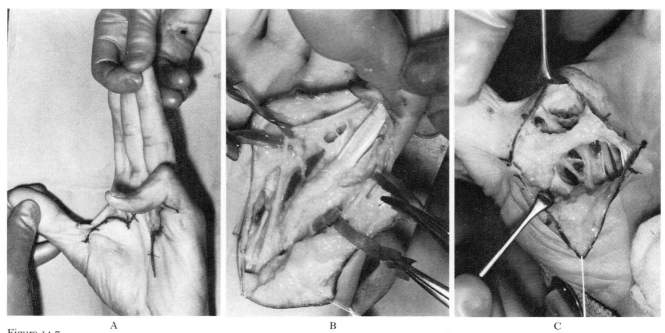

Figure 14.7

A   B   C

A, deformity of the thumb and little finger on the left hand. Formula IP, NP, O, O, 4D%H = 5·5. IP = palmar band at the level of the thumb producing deformity less than 45°. NP = palmar nodules at the base of the index without deformity. O, O = no lesion related to middle or ring finger; 4D+H = Stage 4 deformity of the little finger, i.e., over 135°. Actually one adds the 90° deformity at the PIP to the 30° MP deformity = 120°. If there is no deformity at the distal interphalangeal joint this finger would be coded as = 3. But there is at this DIP level hyperextension deformity H = 45° which is added to the other existing deformities so that 120+35 = 155° = stage 4. The sign + letter D indicates that the deformity is mainly in the finger which implies a worse prognosis than if the deformity were principally the metacarpo-phalangeal joint. 5·5 indicates the total of all the lesions, i.e. thumb = 1; index = 0·5 (N), and little finger = 4.
B, full extension of the PIP joint of the little finger has not been obtained by fasciectomy nor by partial excision of the fibrous flexor sheath which now prevents the use of a skin graft in this region. A Z-plasty was carried out in the skin which happened to be of good quality but if of poor quality some dorsal skin flap may have been necessary to cover the exposed tendons with a secondary free graft to the donor site of the flap.
C, band to the base of the thumb. A Z-plasty in the first web space was not necessary here because the skin was quite supple.

some cases the proximal I.P. joint may have to be immobilized for a few days by an obliquely placed thin Kirschner wire.

SKIN COVERING

Skin cover constitutes one of the key problems in surgical treatment of Dupuytren's contracture. While it comes as the last step in our description of the surgical procedure, it must clearly be taken into account during that the marking out of the skin incision will inevitably influence the mode of closure. Therefore a preoperative assessment of the quantity and quality of skin available must be made. Retracted fibrous tissue, even if it is bulky, will raise no problems if it lies under healthy non-retracted skin, while a flap made out of thickened and poorly vascularized skin is liable to undergo necrosis. The skin must naturally be handled with great care to avoid complications due to poor healing. As much subcutaneous fat as possible should be preserved and the skinflaps and skin edges handled by means of traction threads.

The greatest threat here is skin necrosis with its inevitable sequelae: oedema, delayed mobilization, stiffness. Skin necrosis is frequently due to devascularization of a flap or to wound closure under tension. McCash has shown in fact that it is better to leave a wound unsutured than to have a hematoma trapped under a wound sutured under tension with eventual necrosis.

Necrosis is most likely to occur in the palm where the skin is relatively inelastic and has a poor blood supply in its central part. Besides, palmar complications carry a worse prognosis than digital complications as they can lead to stiffness in healthy fingers. For this very reason, we avoid transposing flaps in the palm if we suspect the slightest risk of necrosis. However, sinuous incisions provide some slight gain in length by sliding the edges during suturing of the skin. Also, as the skin of the hypothenar eminence has a rich blood supply and can be readily mobilized, incisions placed near the ulnar border of the hand will produce some skin gain.

The use of skin grafts in the palm deserve some discussion, they 'take' well enough in the hypothenar region and in the area beyond to the distal palmar crease, as long as the fatty dermal layer persists. However, in the centre of the palm, the exposed tendons following fasciectomy constitute a poor graft bed. Rather than close this area under tension or use flaps of questionable viability, it is probably better to leave the wound partially open and allow spontaneous secondary wound healing. This secondary wound healing is generally quite rapid (several days) as the loss of tegument is usually only in the order of a few millimetres. Rarely is wound healing more troublesome, so long as longitudinal incisions are used and the digital retractions corrected. Occasionally we resort to skin grafts, or in certain cases, we filet a

contracted and functionless finger, usually the 5th, and make use of the skin with its intact neurovascular bundles.

Skin coverage of fingers is a different problem.

Whenever possible we perform a Z-plasty usually based on a midline incision. These plasties are worthwhile and without risk only if certain precautions are taken. When marking out the flaps, one must remember to make angles of not less than 60° and never sharply pointed. The flap must be marked out in ink before the skin is incised. The base of each flap must be freed. Each flap is raised in palmar skin which, as Cleland pointed out in the last century, is separated from the dorsal skin by an osteocutaneous barrier. Rupture of this barrier allows some gain from the looser dorsal skin. It is often necessary and even advisable to do several Z-plasties. The object of the multiple Z-plasties being to borrow from the dorsum in order to lend to the palm; whereas a single Z under tension might produce a stricture. On the other hand, multiple small plasties distribute the gain of dorsal skin over a longer distance and in fact the gain is greater and the risk of stricture is less.

When the teguments appear too unhealthy to tolerate angulated Z-plasties, a rotational flap can be raised from the dorsolateral aspect of the finger. The donor area is then covered with a free graft. Grafts can be resorted to on the palmar aspect of the finger. Even thick grafts have a fair chance of success in this area. They can not be placed directed on the exposed flexor tendons following resection of their fibrous sheath. A combination of grafts and rotated flaps is required to assure coverage which permits the gliding action of the tendons to be maintained. In the rare cases in which the surrounding skin is not suitable for creating flaps, then cross finger flaps or pedicle flaps can be used.

Skin grafts may be performed as a prophylactic measure even when they are not essential for closure. Thus Hueston uses a skin graft at the very first operation in his young patients when clinical findings and etiological factors suggests a tendency to recurrences. But in most cases, the decision to graft is delayed until a recurrence has actually appeared.

Haemostasis. Prevention of postoperative haematomas must remain the surgeon's chief preoccupation. In the course of the dissection, the vessels, depending on their location, must be ligated, if they are close to the pedicle or the skin, or cauterized. When the condition of the patient permits just before letting down the tourniquet, controlled hypotension is useful in that it reduces generalized oozing while allowing coagulation of the residual bleeding points.

Further precautions are application of a compressive dressing, installation of suction drainage for 48 hours and systematic checking of the dressing on the second postoperative day for evacuation of an eventual haematoma.

Postoperative care. A plaster slab on the back of the forearm and hand immobilizes the wrist in extension and the M.P. joints in about 30° of flexion so as to avoid traction on the palmar sutures.

The position of immobilization for the I.P. joints deserves some mention. If retraction at these joints is relatively limited, say less than 50°, and if complete correction has been easily achieved, the joints may be left free to move within the cast. If however, retraction was long standing and severe, it is better to keep the I.P. joints extended. In those cases where muscular contracture tends to reproduce the deformity, the joints may be immobilized for a few days with Kirschner wires.

The arm is suspended for 48 hours; the patient is allowed to go home on the third day with instructions to actively mobilize all the joints in the limb which have been left free.

Plaster cast and Kirschner wires are removed after a week. Depending on the condition of the wound, the hand may be left exposed or may be covered with a light dressing which allows physiotherapy. At first flexion exercises are encouraged as they do not produce traction on the wound, then extension movements are then started gradually. At the first sign of oedema, the patient is told to keep his arm elevated between the sessions of physiotherapy. If the oedema persists, the patient should be readmitted to the ward for a few days so as to supervise the position of the limb and mobilization of the fingers, and to prevent the development of chronic oedema.

The skin sutures are taken out late, between the second and third week, as healing in the palm is slow. When skin healing is complete, active steps must be taken to combat residual retractions with the help of posture braces worn between sessions of physiotherapy, and later only at night. In patients who have had a fasciotomy, we fit the hand in a dorsal elastic traction brace to extend the fingers immediately after the operation.

To conclude we would like again to stress the importance of surgical technique in the treatment of Dupuytren's contracture. We are convinced that, while they cannot guarantee satisfactory results in every case, meticulous surgery combined with close postoperative supervision by the surgeon himself have a considerable influence on the quality of these results.

15. TECHNIQUE OF SELECTIVE APONEURECTOMY FOR DUPUYTREN'S CONTRACTURE

Julian M. Bruner

The successful treatment of Dupuytren's disease must begin with the careful selection of patients who may be expected to benefit from surgery, and the rejection of others. The purpose of treatment is to relieve joint contracture by removing hyperplastic fascia in the distal palm and in the affected digits.

Total aponeurectomy has been abandoned because of complications and protracted disability. Fasciotomy and amputation of a hopeless digit are useful palliative measures in some cases. The definitive treatment of choice is limited aponeurectomy.

Aponeurectomy is limited to that fascia which is hyperplastic at the time of surgery. It is especially directed to those longitudinal bands which bridge the joints and to other bands which exist in relation to transverse stresses in the hand, notably in the distal palm near the base of the ring finger.

The surgeon should resect the hyperplastic fascia and nothing but the fascia. Fat should not be removed, and the three colliculi in the distal palm should remain intact.

Technical considerations are of prime importance and will be discussed under the following headings: incision, haemostasis, magnification, instrumentation, wound closure. The points to be mentioned are not new, but are stressed because these middle aged and elderly hands are especially vulnerable to surgical trauma, which therefore must be minimized.

1. INCISION

The traditional long transverse incision in the distal palm is no longer used. Although it results in a favourable scar cosmetically, this is almost its only virtue. Exposure of the underlying pretendinous fascial bands is poor, and there is danger of wound dehiscence from early postoperative motion of the M.P. joints. Worst of all, the resulting deep transverse scar seems to form a coffer-dam against afferent tissue fluids, resulting in protracted swelling of the distal plam and fingers.

A longitudinal zig-zag incision is now preferred. It gives excellent exposure, heals readily without contracture, and permits early motion of the hand. It causes less oedema because it obstructs fewer venous and lymphatic channels.

The exact incision is delineated before tourniquet pressure is applied. It is 'tailor-made' for each case, and no two hands are alike. If there is only one longitudinal palmar band causing contracture, the incision criss-crosses this band. If there are two bands, the incision may oscillate between the two. But if two parallel incision are made, they must not be contiguous, or blood supply of the skin may be compromised. The palmar incision may be continued distally over the involved digit, with a transverse component over the M.P. joint, or a narrow bridge of skin may be left.

The angles at the hinges of the incision are important. Obtuse angles may be used safely with skin of poor quality, but acute angles pose a real risk of slow healing or actual slough. If, in addition, pointed skin flaps are to be transposed as in Z-plasty in which acute angles of 60° are inherent, that risk is increased.

Therefore Z-plasty which gains a little length, should be reserved for use in those cases where the skin is of good quality locally. It is most useful in the digits at joint level, and is never used in the palm.

2. HAEMOSTASIS

Perfect haemostasis during operation is essential for safe and rapid aponeurectomy. The hand is simply elevated before tourniquet pressure is applied. Preliminary exsanguination of the hand is a disadvantage. Some blood remaining in the vessels aids in their identification.

During tourniquet ischaemia of the hand, heat is harmful because it increases tissue reaction. Saline solutions for wound irrigation should be cold, not warm. Hot spot-lights may also damage ischemic tissues.

3. MAGNIFICATION

A 2x magnifying loupe is routinely used during the dissection. The differentiation of fine strands of fascia from fine nerves and blood vessels is thereby facilitated. Injury of digital nerves is completely avoidable, because they can be plainly seen.

Such low power magnification provides a focal depth of 3 inches, with a working distance of 10 inches, which gives ample scope for the manoeuvers of aponeurectomy. Also it does not require the use of more powerful lights such as those used for microsurgery.

4. INSTRUMENTATION

The ordinary instruments of general surgery are not suitable for aponeurectomy. A small scalpel is used for transecting heavy fascial bands and for separating skin from fascia, but much of the dissection should be done with curved, blunt-pointed iris scissors. Skin margins are retracted with fine skin hooks. Tendons and nerves are held aside with button hook retractors. Thus surgical trauma is minimized.

5. WOUND CLOSURE

At the end of operation, which is usually completed within one hour, tourniquet pressure is released, the hand elevated and pressure applied to the wound. If aponeurectomy has been done as above, there is usually little if any active bleeding (if bleeding points are present, they are tied with fine gut).

There will be some oozing however in all cases. Therefore routine drainage of the wound is essential and will effectively prevent hematoma. The retention of bloody serum within the wound is harmful.

The skin is closed with 4-0 nylon sutures, and one or two gum rubber drains 5 mm in diameter are placed at strategic points to be removed in 48 hours.

Attention to these five technical points will reduce the trauma of aponeurectomy in these elderly hands, minimize complications, and permit early motion of the hand, so essential to full recovery.

16. SOME PRACTICAL POINTS IN THE SURGICAL TREATMENT OF DUPUYTREN'S CONTRACTURE

Mortimer Shaw

Although the cause of Dupuytren's contracture remains a mystery, the results of treatment have improved in recent years. The improvement may be attributed in part to the general acceptance of the principles of atraumatic hand surgery, with the consequent acceleration of healing with minimal tissue reaction. Increase in knowledge has been disseminated by the activities of National Hand Clubs and international meetings, where the stimulus of discussion has arisen between those who have a special interest in the relief of deformity from an orthopaedic standpoint, and those specially interested in plastic repair. Attention has been directed to the fallacy of employing any single routine method in every case, and to the disastrous results which may follow an extensive resection under unsuitable conditions. Care has been taken to diminish the number and consequences of complications and a selective approach to treatment has been widely adopted. I propose to refer briefly to five points where experience has shown the need for a careful selective assessment of individual cases.

I. ADAPTING THE EXTENT OF THE SURGERY TO ACCORD WITH INDIVIDUAL FACTORS IN THE PATIENT

The proper extent of surgical interference may be limited firstly by general conditions now well recognized. These include old age, alcoholism, and a constitutional tendency to swell. Secondly, by local defects in the hand itself, such as joint disorder, vasomotor dysfunction and trophic change in the skin. In the absence of these two factors the deformity should be released as thoroughly as the joint and tendon sheath contractures will allow.

2. SELECTING THE SURGICAL APPROACH TO CONFORM WITH THE DISTRIBUTION OF THE DISEASED FASCIA

As in any other surgical condition adequate open exposure is necessary to perform a delicate excision. This requires a mainly longitudinal incision which, however, has to be modified at the beginning or at the end of the operation in order to avoid subsequent contracture inherent in such an incision. Z flaps may be raised at the start if this helps the exposure, or they may be designed at the end of the procedure, often more effectively, when the skin shortage is apparent. The approach may need to be single, duplicated, or even triplicated in the same hand when there is widespread involvement of the fascia, as has been described so beautifully by Raoul Tubiana. The more one appreciates the advantages of longitudinal extensile incisions, the less one employs the transverse incision.

The latter is statistically more liable to the complications of haematoma, loss of skin, and delayed healing. A zig-zag incision in the palm, without transposing the flaps, is the most generally useful and dependable.

3. SELECTING THE EXTENT OF FASCIAL RESECTION

When one has experienced the rigidity and the complexity of the contracted bands found at operation one can appreciate the extent of dissection which may be needed before improvement in contracture is obtained. A contracted central band of palmar fascia causing flexion at the metacarpophalangeal joint can often be seen before the incision is made, and it may be easy to eradicate; but the deeply placed contracted lateral bands firmly anchored to tendon sheaths, deep fascia, and bone, are often unsuspected until the exposure is made, and it may require great patience and dexterity to remove them without damaging the important structures in the palm. Thus the need to widen the scope of the procedure is often only apparent at the time of the operation. Similarly, the adhesions to the skin may be such as to require rather extended dissection, and removal of the 'natatory ligaments' in the interdigital webs, may be necessary to free the lateral contracture and widen the span of the hand. It is therefore just as illogical to speak of a routine limited band excision as of a routine radical excision, and we speak instead of a 'limited' or 'wide' resection according to the needs of the case. The excision is concerned with a block of fascia including a margin of the macroscopically normal fascia on each side. Too narrow an excision may be followed by early recurrence. On the other hand one tries to avoid unnecessary stripping of vessels and nerves and the removal of fatty tissues, in order to limit the dead space left behind in the palm after the resection. This unforeseen need to extend the procedure dictates a flexible and extensile approach, and requires ingenuity and experience in the subsequent skin repair.

4. SELECTING THE SKIN CLOSURE

When the contracture has been improved the skin

of the palm and of the fingers will be short, especially in the long axis. This may be due to infiltration of the skin by the disease process itself, with a loss of the subdermal fatty layer. The nutritional state of the skin will dictate the size and situation of any transposed Z flaps. Most of the gain in extension has taken place in the fingers rather than in the palm, and the Z plasty, single or multiple, is most effective at finger level, quite apart from its virtue in providing the most perfect exposure. The transposition of Z flaps in the palm, however, is less satisfactory, the skin flaps being thicker, and stiffer and inelastic. It is preferable to accept the skin shortage in the palm in the interests of early quick healing and to rely upon the gradual natural improvement as the skin regains its elasticity with use and resolution of deep scar. An immediate free graft in the palm is not advisable since it tends to delay the resumption of activity and because it adds a hazard to the deeper structures if it fails. Even if it succeeds, it contributes a sensory deficiency to the palm.

5. SELECTION OF THE MODE OF AFTER CARE

The dead space below the undermined area requires to be gently obliterated by apposition of the skin flaps to the deeper dissection, in order to avoid the serious complication of haematoma. This object is often most successively achieved by the use of continuous suction at a negative pressure of 10–15 cm of mercury, maintained by a suction pump acting through a plastic catheter. This provides a negative pressure limited to the dead space, without the need for additional pressure from outside on the undermined skin, other than that provided by the pressure of the atmosphere. The method also avoids dorsal and lateral compression of the hand.

Sponge and other soft dressings and crepe bandages can also be successful, but the suction method allows the added advantage of early exposure of the hand skin to the light and air which aids healing by providing a dry cool wound. Exposure interferes least of all with gentle active interphalangeal movements. The wrist is immobilized in dorsiflexion by a dorsal plaster slab while the suction is in use. The slab limits extension of the metacarpophalangeal joints, so that the palmar skin is relaxed, but allows interphalangeal movements to take place. The hand is elevated for 48 hours.

The suction catheter can be intermittently clamped and disconnected from the pump in order to allow the patient to be mobile, but is usually retained for 4 days. Because of the need for early use of the fingers, some of the stitches are retained for two weeks. Dressings are kept to a minimum. Restoration of hand and finger movements is a natural function associated with little discomfort or oedema, and physiotherapy is limited to supervision of the active purposeful finger movements and their gradual increase, and to the insistence upon shoulder exercises from the beginning. Complications supervene at times, as in all surgical endeavours, but their consequences can be minimised if they are anticipated in every case and discovered by careful inspection in the first 48 hours. Prompt evacuation of a haematoma at this early stage with a renewal of the suction can prevent long standing discomfort and disability. The most important guiding principle is the recognition that although treatment is directed to a relief of the contracture by the restoration of lost extension of the digits, this aim shall always take second place to that of maintaining a strong, full, supple, painless grip of the hand.

17. SPECIAL POINTS OF TECHNIQUE IN DUPUYTREN'S CONTRACTURE

J. W. Littler

Few afflictions of the hand have received more attention than the palmar and digital fascial contracture described by Dupuytren. The aetiologic confusion of this fourth to fifth decade fibrous metaplasia persists, but advanced surgical techniques can afford relief for many disabled hands.

The distressing operative morbidity probably parallels closely (or surpasses) that of untreated cases. Realistically speaking, the functional and economic loss following surgery has been so great that most surgeons abhor the thought of any radical attack. The many stiffened joints, necrosed palms, severed digital nerves, lend poignant support to the thesis of non-intervention. Nevertheless, carefully performed, a resection of the involved palmar and digital fascia can afford great relief for serious disability. The foremost requirement is a rational selection of cases for a fascial resection or a subcutaneous palmar division. The lesion is not urgent, and it seems feasible to allow some progression rather than to recommend intervention the moment a nodule appears or the palmar skin is retracted at one point. The recent proposal that early excision of only the palmar nodule or plaque stems the development of a contracture may have merit, but the disease is unpredictable and can develop elsewhere. Assurance of the benign nature of the process, progressive though it is generally relieves the patient of undue anxiety.

When, however, hypertrophy and contracture of the fascia limits finger extension at the metacarpophalangeal and or proximal interphalangeal levels, the operation is indicated before the skin is severely compromised. The palm and digit pose two contrasting regions with respect to ease of fascial excision and prediction of the result. The palmar dissection is less complicated than the fingers and whereas metacarpophalangeal release is the rule, restoration of extension at the proximal interphalangeal joints often is not realised. The close relationship of the fascia to the dermis is such that surgical separation can be extremely difficult in advanced cases, and may occasionally necessitate excision of involved skin and the use of a free thick skin graft to complete coverage. Brachial plexus block analgesia is highly satisfactory for the procedure, and the pneumatic tourniquet is mandatory.

The dissection can be one of the most difficult known to the hand surgeon, and it is definitely not for the tyro. Certain fascial distributions demand special incisions for adequate exposure, yet these must be so designed that they will permit healing without secondary scar contracture or skin loss (Figs. 17.1, 17.2, 17.3). In more advanced cases, involving the proximal aspect of the digit, a Z-plasty (as recommended by McIndoe) is

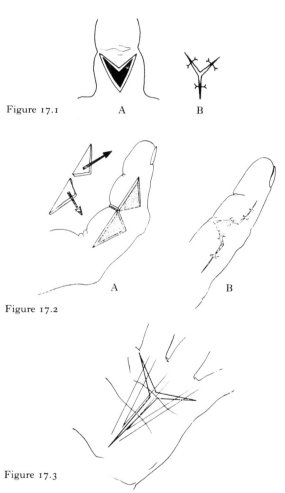

Figure 17.1   A   B

Figure 17.2   A   B

Figure 17.3

of value for good exposure and a gain in skin length but only if the proximal interphalangeal joint has not undergone secondary contracture. Exquisite care is required to separate the two skin flaps from the underlying fascia and yet retain their circulation. When the proximal interphalangeal joint is restrained in flexion by contracted fascia and skin the limbs of the Z can be made at an angle of approximately 80 degrees (rather than the usual 60 degrees), for with the resection of the restraining fascia the joint release opens the proximal segment and allows the two flaps to alternate and fall into position. Furthermore, the skin is tented abnormally by the bowstringing fascia, and the use of a Z incision takes advantage of this increase. Unfortunately, the proximal

interphalangeal joint, secondarily altered by an intrinsic contracture, flexor tendon and sheath fixation is not always relieved by the fascial resection. This is especially true of the little finger. An interesting observation in a large series of fascial resections is that a free skin graft was rarely needed, but the Z-plasty was often used at the digit base (Fig. 17.4). Digital recurrences may

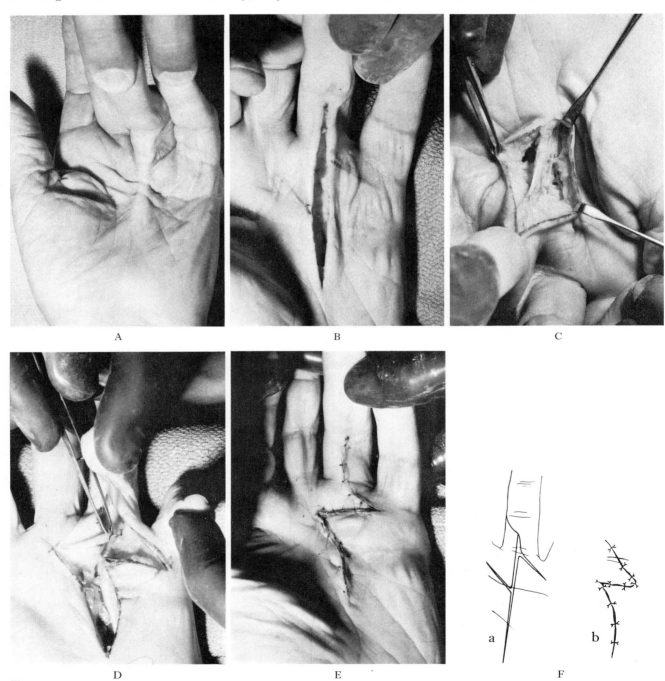

Figure 17.4
Incision is commenced at the base of the finger and the skin margins lengthened by Z-plasty.

require secondary excision of skin and fascia and the use of a full-thickness graft. A distant pedicle graft has been required only in a referred case in which, following an operation, the palmar skin necrosed and secondary healing led to a critical contracture. At all costs, hand function must not be jeopardized by the urge to excise the thickened fascia at the expense of crucial skin.

Palmar skin is nourished by vertical branches originating from the neurovascular bundles coursing deep between the longitudinal fibres of the pretendinous bands and roofed at the metacarpophalangeal levels by the transverse fibres. Diseased fascia in an advanced state is drawn to the overlying dermis through a contracture of the fasciodermal fibres, the normal intervening fat is lost, and skin and fascia become one, making separation difficult, at times impossible, and skin survival precarious. Fortunately, only limited areas are generally severely involved, and nourishment is assured, especially if one or more of the vertical vessels can be preserved. The resection is made more difficult, but the result satisfies the effort.

Once the abnormal fascia has been completely exposed, its vertical septa are isolated (with care for the lumbrical and neurovascular systems) and divided at the level of the deep fascia and intermetacarpal ligaments. Abnormally heavy septal extensions pass from the pretendinous bands bilaterally to the fibrous tendon sheath just distal to the intermetacarpal* ligament, where they envelop the interosseous tendons and pass dorsally into the extensor hood. Traction on these yoke-like septa can flex the metacarpophalangeal joint. Preservation of the synovial cul-de-sac is precarious at this point where the heavy septa from the pretendinous bands encircle the proximal aspect of the fibrous tendon sheath. The relationship of the pretendinous band and its yoke to the tendon sheath is somewhat like that of the superficialis tendon to the profundus. An attempt must be made not to open the intact synovial sheaths, because blood within them produces discomfort, voluntary immobilization and possibly stiffened fingers. The encircling fibres prevent metacarpophalangeal release when the pretendinous band alone is sectioned just distal to them at the metacarpophalangeal level in the operation known as subcutaneous fasciotomy. Prolongation of the pretendinous bands into the proximal phalanx is generally more to one side. In the fifth digit the fascia also arises as a prolongation from the common tendon of insertion of the intrinsic abductor and flexor muscles (Fig. 17.5), or flexor sheath bridges the proximal interphalangeal joint, and inserts into the fibrous tendon sheath and extensor mechanism.

The relationship of the neurovascular bundle to the fibrous extension is critical for at the palmardigital level it often passes superficial and mesial to the band,

* Inter volar plate.

and deep and lateral to it at the proximal interphalangeal level. Variations are not exceptional. Great care must be exercised during the fascial resection not to damage this important vascular and tactile link. Whereas division of the pretendinous band can be made at the metacarpophalangeal level where it bowstrings the joint high above the deep laterally lying neurovascular bundles, such a division is fraught with disaster within the digit, where through possible encirclement the two are intimately combined.

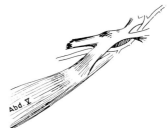

Figure 17.5

The fact that extension gained at the time of the fascial resection cannot be maintained when the contracted skin is closed is not of immediate concern. The chief factors are the resection of the involved fascia with preservation of viable skin and the gaining of primary healing with the hand in good functional position. Active metacarpophalangeal flexion and extension exercises can be started about three weeks postoperatively when all dressing support is removed. It is unnecessary for the early postoperative patient to practice vigorous hand activity, for if the synovial sheaths of the digit have not been entered they will be free of haemorrhagic irritation, and active interphalangeal movement will be possible and painless even early with the hand immobilized in a dressing supported by a plaster shell. Maintenance of the transverse and longitudinal arches of the hand with the wrist in extension and the metacarpophalangeal joints in some flexious, to ease the skin closure, is essential following the fascial excision.

Early unsupported activity causes swelling and induration of the unhealed palmar tissues. Dressing support for 3 to 4 weeks has been found eminently successful in preventing this complication. Immediate postoperative suction of the palm for the control of any bleeding, has been advocated by Barron and others. Haematoma is a rarity with good haemostasis, careful dissection and closure, and support of the palm by an anterior–posterior compression dressing and plaster shell. Furthermore, the necessary control of haemorrhage forces preoperative attention to the possibility of an altered clotting mechanism in the Dupuytren patient through a check of liver function and of bleeding and clotting time. At the end of a 4 week period of immobilization the best treatment appears to be the use of silicone putty as an exercise medium for a progressive return of a more normal supple hand.

18. OPERATIVE DIFFICULTIES AND POSTOPERATIVE COMPLICATIONS IN THE SURGERY OF DUPUYTREN'S CONTRACTURE

J. Michon

Certain difficulties may arise at different stages in the surgical treatment of Dupuytren's contracture and we should be aware of these in order to anticipate and overcome them if the occasion should arise.

Postoperative complications early or late equally merit our serious consideration. Some complications are directly related to the operative technique and thus become a moral responsibility, if not a medicolegal one. Others on the contrary are quite unpredictable, but they all must be constantly borne in mind if we are to lessen their consequences.

OPERATIVE DIFFICULTIES

PLANNING THE INCISION

For several years we have used the angled digito-palmar incisions which have been elaborated by Tubiana. This has produced a considerable improvement in our results with a reduction in the incidence and severity of skin necrosis. Moreover when necrosis does occur it does not interrupt the postoperative active mobilization of the hand which otherwise would put dangerous traction on the suture line.

The planning of these longitudinal incisions, which can be adapted with precision to each case must obey certain rules.

(a) With pen and ink we first of all mark the areas of skin fixation and dimpling in the distal palm, as well as the bands and nodules to be excised, so as to ensure that the skin flaps when raised will have the safest blood supply. The incision is then drawn to pass through the most adherent areas and as close as possible to the skin dimples, while at the same time allowing adequate exposure of the underlying lesions without excessive undermining of the skin margins.

(b) If several fingers are involved only one of the digital incisions should be extended into the palm.

(c) If previous scarring in the area is so gross or extensive as to endanger the circulation of the local skin flaps, some plans should be prepared for its excision should the need arise. If the fibrous sheath of the flexor tendons can be retained intact the skin defect can then be made good by a thick split skin graft or a full thickness graft (Hueston, 1969). If, however, the fibrous flexor sheath has been opened or excised a rotation flap will be necessary, particularly on the finger. We prefer a clas-

sical rotation flap on the same finger and only use the cross finger flap on the extremely rare occasions in the correction of Dupuytren's contracture.

(d) Figure 1 shows some examples of excisions adapted to particular cases. It is in fact impossible to lay down a strict set of rules since cases vary and we need an open and imaginative mind in such an area where nothing can replace experience (Figs. 18.1, 18.2).

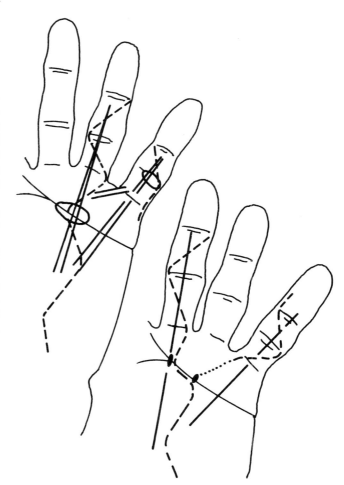

Figure 18.1
Some examples of incisions used for exposure and capable of adaptation to the distribution of the major lesions. Areas of likely skin adherence are shown by circles and skin pits by dots.

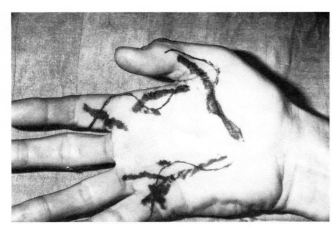

Figure 18.2
Extensive Dupuytren's disease where only the middle finger was not involved. Three incisions allowed adequate clearance.

DISSECTION AND RESECTION

It cannot be stated too often that the dissection must be centred on the nerves. But it is equally important to emphasize the need to preserve the arteries which may be less easily defined but which are probably responsible for a considerable number of postoperative skin necroses and late trophic disturbances.

The anatomy of the bands and nodules is now well established, having been clarified by the recent studies of Tubiana *et al.* and J. Gosset to name only the French workers. We only wish to point out here the importance of the nodule on the medial aspect of the metacarpophalangeal joint of the little finger, closely applied to the tendon of abductor digiti minimi and involved from the beginning with the dorsolateral aponeurosis of finger. This concept of the local anatomy of this nodule is the key to adequate correction of the two proximal joints of the little finger.

FIXED FLEXION DEFORMITIES

The anatomy of the capsule and ligaments of the metacarpophalangeal joint clearly explains why there is never any difficulty in obtaining full extension at this level after fasciectomy.

On the contrary, when P.I.P. flexion deformity exceeds 90 degrees (stage IIID and IVD) fasciectomy alone often fails to give satisfactory passive extension of the finger.

The flexion deformity seems to be fixed by several factors:

1. Longitudinal contraction of the fibrous flexor sheath. Simply incising the sheath longitudinally is often not enough and it may be necessary to carry out a veritable synovectomy with excision particularly of the volar plate of the P.I.P. joint.

2. Fixation and contracture of the volar plate: the best method of release is that of Curtis (1966), excision of plate through two lateral exposures (Fig. 18.3).

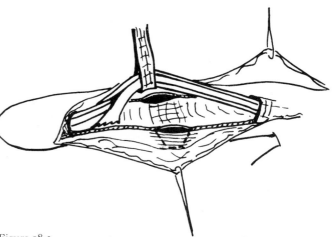

Figure 18.3
Arthrolysis of the proximal interphalangeal joint according to Curtis, i.e., resection of the synovial sheath, glenoid ligament and, if necessary, lateral capsulectomy.

3. Contracture of the collateral ligaments: it may be necessary to perform bilateral capsulectomy if simple palmar clearance is not enough to provide complete extension.

4. The interosseus and extensor apparatus: even after tendon and joint release procedures it is often found that, although full passive extension is possible, the flexion deformity relentlessly recurs when the finger is released. The similarity to a boutonniere deformity is striking.

If the boutonniere deformity is normally due to a tendon lesion with secondary joint changes, the present situation in D.C. seems to be the reverse, in that the joint deformity produces secondarily a palmar luxation of the lateral bands of the extensor apparatus and a progressive stretching of the median band with sometimes even a contracture of Landsmeer's retinacular ligament.

A secondary factor must be added, namely that in several cases we have been able to demonstrate a volar adhesion of the interosseous tendon on the dorsolabinal aspect of the metacarpophalangeal joint. At the level of the metacarpal neck, invasion of one of Kanavel's septa can produce a large nodule which can effectively fix the origin of the interosseus tendon against the skeleton (Fig. 18.4). Surgical dissection of tendon at this level can avoid actually sectioning it or its expansion at P.I.P. level. It may be necessary to shorten the triangular ligament by two or three sutures at P.I.P. level.

Plication to tighten the middle slip of the extensor

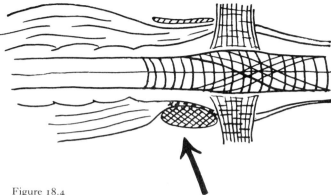

Figure 18.4
A deep nodule producing interference with interosseous excursion at the region of the metacarpophalangeal joint and requiring incision of the deep fascia here to free the intrinsic tendon.

tendon is not essential in the re-establishment of extensor tendon function and its tone will usually recover with use of the conventional splints and postoperative physiotherapy.

SKIN CLOSURE AND PLASTIC PROBLEMS

Since we have been using the digitopalmar incision we have had far less need for plastic procedures at the end of the operation. When the blood supply of the skin looks as though it may be precarious we plan a sinuous incision, eliminating the sharp angles of the zig-zag. During wound closure the sinuosities flatten out and allow some lengthening effect, particularly useful in cases with severe flexion deformity (Fig. 18.5A).

When the angles of the zig-zag have been preserved in its usual form, short transverse incisions opposite these points of the sharp flaps allow a natural lengthening effect which is most effective in the M.P. and P.I.P. zones (Fig. 18.5B).

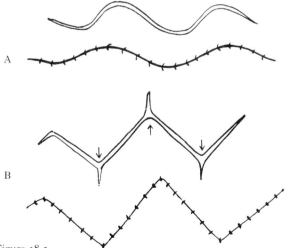

Figure 18.5
A, Lengthening obtained from a sinuous incision because of elasticity of the skin; B, Lengthening obtained from a zig zag incision by deepening of each angle.

As already stated, we tend more and more to excise skin devitalized by the dissection and to replace these areas by free grafts or flaps. A useful assessment of the viability in doubtful areas of skin can be obtained by watching the return of colour after temporary release of the tourniquet (Fig. 18.6).

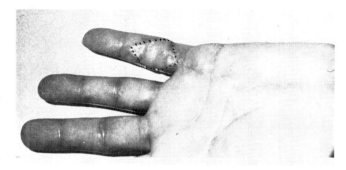

Figure 18.6
Full thickness skin graft to the little finger carried out at the time of fasciectomy is quite stable by 6 weeks.

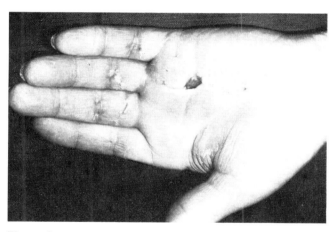

Figure 18.7
Postoperative skin necrosis in the palm which healed with only minimum scar contracture. Note that the zig-zag exposure has allowed active mobilisation despite this complication.

POSTOPERATIVE COMPLICATIONS

1. PALMAR HAEMATOMA

This was relatively frequent with the transverse incision of McIndoe and we have already markedly reduced this incision by use of continuous suction (Redon) using a perforated intravenous catheter No. 4.

Since using longitudinal incisions haematoma has become quite exceptional but we still use continuous palmar suction during the first three postoperative days. Occasionally, however, we find a later serous collection in the palm which can be easily evacuated by removing a suture and applying firm pressure on one or two occasions.

2. SKIN IRRITATION

Skin irritation around the wound margins has also been virtually eliminated since the composition of the greasy commercial wound dressing has been modified. In any case this minor complication has always rapidly cleared up with some local corticoid creams.

3. SKIN NECROSIS

We have already indicated the means of preventing skin necrosis:
(a) Careful design of skin incisions.
(b) Preservation of digital arteries and their collateral branches during dissection of the fascia.
(c) Excision of doubtfully viable areas of skin.

Nevertheless skin necrosis remains the most frequent of our complications. It usually is seen as a round or oval slough over the proximal phalangeal segment near its base or near the distal palmar creaseline.

If the slough is no wider than 1 centimetre it separates by the fifteenth day and spontaneously heals. Its most serious sequel is a hypertrophic scar which is occasionally mildly contracted (Fig. 18.7).

However, if the skin deficit reaches or exceeds 1 centimetre, healing is likely to be much slower, possibly associated with deep infection and at best will leave a scar contracture sufficient to interfere with normal finger function. It is thus essential to excise the slough as soon as possible and to repair the defect by a free graft or rotation flap along the lines already laid down for these two procedures (Fig. 18.8).

It is obvious that, if skin necrosis occurs in a finger already grossly handicapped from long-standing flexion deformity, the final result is likely to be so poor that early amputation may have to be considered (Fig. 9).

Acute Ischaemic Necrosis of the Finger. After attempting correction of a little finger flexed to stage IV we have twice encountered digital ischaemic necrosis. In one case it was obvious that the two digital arteries had been injured during the operation. In the other case the finger had been splinted postoperatively with the proximal interphalangeal joint in excessive extension so that postoperative thrombosis was precipitated. Naturally these two complications required early amputation of the necrotic digits.

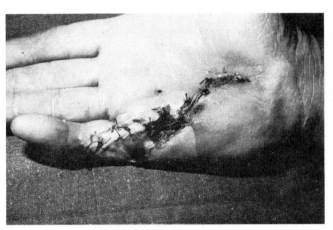

Figure 18.9
Serious postoperative skin necrosis attributed to division of the medial digital vessel to the little finger. Amputated on the 6th day.

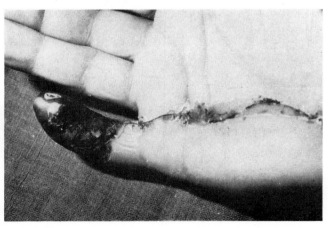

Figure 18.10
Necrosis of the little finger attributed to the postoperative dressing forcing the finger into extension too rapidly.

Postoperative Trophic Disturbances and Physiotherapy.
Oedema is probably one of the most commonly encountered postoperative phenomena after surgery for Dupuytren's contracture. Usually it is only temporary, appearing after the fourth day and disappearing about

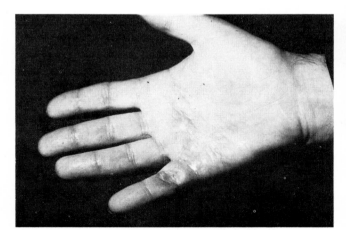

Figure 18.8
Postoperative skin necrosis in the little finger treated by excision and skin grafting on the 5th day. The result at 6 weeks is shown.

the time when active movements are resumed, about the twentieth day. However, in some cases it assumes a more severe form and lasts longer, becoming then a serious handicap to the recovery of full hand movements. Sudek's atrophy is probably the most severe complication after surgery for Dupuytren's contracture (Fig. 18.11). Its onset is to be suspected when a severe oedema phase is associated with a painful tension in the hand and with more or less severe aches spasmodically extending into the fingers.

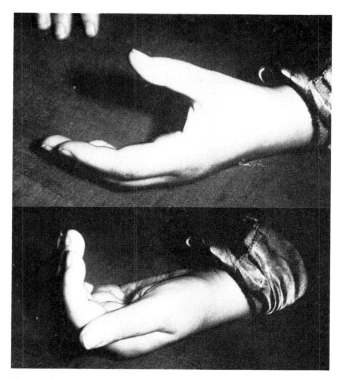

Figure 18.11
Sudek's atrophy in a rheumatic patient showing the range of movement at 3 months and requiring up to 2 years for recovery of normal movement.

The aetiology of this painful postoperative dystrophy remains a mystery. A recent American study (Stein, 1962) showed an interesting association between Sudek's syndrome and the common median nerve compression in the carpal tunnel and it has been proposed that routine decompression of the median nerve be an early measure to be taken in Sudek's syndrome. We have carried this out on three patients with postoperative pain after fasciectomy—one patient operated on by us, two referred after operation elsewhere—and in these three cases the relief of pain has been rapid and the oedema has markedly decreased in a few days allowing resumption of the normal postoperative routine. Although no final conclusion on aetiology can be drawn

from this, the value of this decompression is very real and we believe that this simple, rapid and safe procedure should be done routinely at the slightest warning of the onset of Sudek's atrophy.

If we are operating on patients whom we suspect to be predisposed to trophic and vascular disturbances we now routinely decompress the carpal tunnel at the end of the fasciectomy. This applies to patients with acute or chronic rheumatic disorders in the hand or cervical spondylitis as well as those with numbness of the fingers at night or unexplained pains in the hands. The six patients so far treated this way have all had a straightforward postoperative functional recovery.

A physiotherapist is not usually necessary after correction of mild cases who have had only early flexion deformity. But in more severe cases and whenever joint stiffness threatens at 15 to 20 days a period of supervised re-education under a competent physiotherapist is absolutely essential. Daily active movement of the fingers, joint by joint, is assisted by very gentle passive movements—but the active movements by the patient himself are by far the most important part of this regime.

A gentle traction splint using elastics, or better still springs (Iselin), is essential as well as the physiotherapy, whenever capsulectomies have been necessary in the correction of the flexion deformity. This splint is worn almost continuously in the early stages and then each night for several months later (Fig. 18.12).

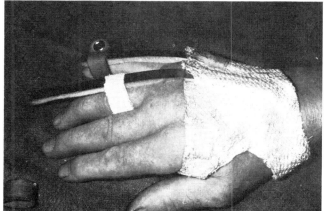

Figure 18.12
Spring splint for postoperative extension (Iselin).

RESULTS AND RECURRENCES

Follow-up studies of long series have made it clear for some time now that operation on early stages of the disease will ensure recovery of a normally functional hand, both in extension and flexion, while it is clear that operation on advanced cases (stages III and IV) is less often followed by complete functional recovery. Even if in severe cases full extension is obtained at operation it is not uncommon for some degree of P.I.P. flexion deformity to persist. This deformity is due to capsular contracture and associated deep scarring. In some particularly unfortunate cases this loss of flexion is also associated with a loss of active flexion due also to peri-articular fibrosis or adhesions of the flexor tendons (Fig. 18.13).

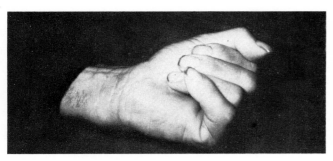

Figure 18.13
Loss of flexion after proximal interphalangeal arthrolysis (3rd degree digital deformity in a chronic rheumatic patient; note the knuckle pads).

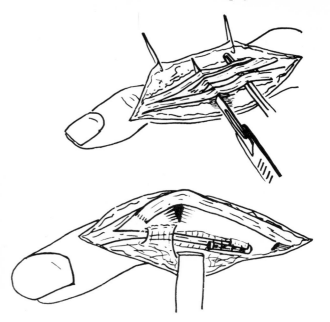

Figure 18.14
Tenolysis of the extensor apparatus, dorsal capsulotomy and a Littler tenodesis to correct the Swan neck deformity.

In some particularly severe cases we see a rapid or progressive stiffness of the fingers, usually the little finger, which become fixed in a more or less severe flexion at P.I.P. level with extension at D.I.P. level while the M.P. joint remains mobile.

Rarely we have seen, after a painful swollen post-operative phase, an intrinsic plus type of deformity, which becomes fixed in a few weeks with the finger held in varying degrees of swan-neck deformity. This is a particularly vicious complication since it prevents finger flexion and prehensile activity of the hand and can only be corrected by dorsolateral capsulectomies of the P.I.P. joints and construction of a Littler type tenodesis to prevent recurrence of hyperextension at this level (Figs. 18.14, 18.15).

The quality of the operative scars is determined not only by the presence or absence of delayed wound healing but equally by the preoperative state of the skin. If the skin retains its suppleness and a good layer of subcutaneous fibrofatty tissue the scar will be fine and often almost invisible. If, on the other hand, the skin has been dissected only with difficulty from the underlying pathological tissue it is going to behave more or less as a free graft during the healing phase and will become fixed to the deeper structures. Frequently these areas become hypertrophic and contracted with all the more risk of some necrosis, even slight, slowing up final healing.

Apart from wound healing problems there is occasionally seen after a period of palmar oedema a particularly indurated subcutaneous fibrous plaque in the centre of the palm.

In all these complications, hypertrophy, contraction or fibrosis, we have found a prolonged course of iodized ionization to be the best method of minimizing the late consequences of these unpleasant complications.

True recurrences must not be confused with early return of the preoperative flexion deformity nor with extension of the disease process outside the zone cleared by fasciectomy. One can only speak of recurrence when

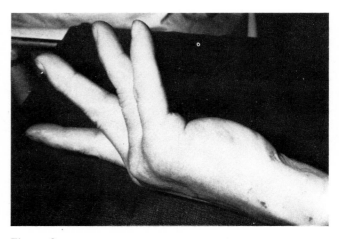

Figure 18.15
Postoperative state in a patient with predominantly palmar lesion and a predisposition to swan neck deformity.

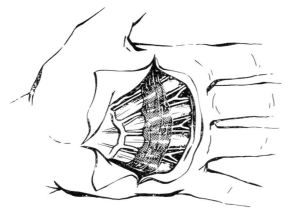

Figure 19.2

Diagram showing the transverse palmar ligament after removal of the longitudinal pretendinous bands. This ligament is never the site of pathological lesions indicative of Dupuytren's disease.

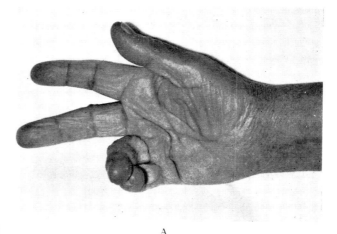

A

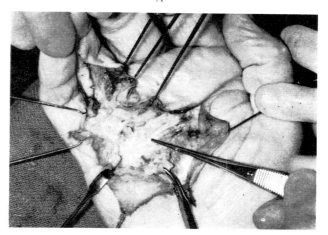

B

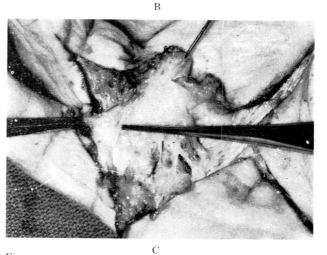

C

characteristics; this despite the personal experience at that time in removing the palmar aponeurosis for the treatment of Dupuytren's contracture in about 400 hands. The explanation why this constant structure was overlooked is the operative technique that had been used, i.e. the palmar aponeurosis was severed transversely in the proximal part of the palm and the alternate tunnels for flexor tendons and nerves, vessels, and lumbricals were split open by longitudinal incisions; the sections thus isolated were excised by cutting the paratendinous septa. With this technique the transverse palmar ligament never became exposed.

In marked contrast to the characteristic behaviour of the transverse fibres in the palmar region, the interdigital ligaments are frequently the site of pathological changes, resulting in contracted bands which prevent the fingers from being separated (Fig. 19.3). The fibre bundles of normal interdigital ligaments are, however, in character indistinguishable from those which form the transverse ligament in the palm.

PATHOGENESIS

Since Dupuytren first described the deformity as produced by contraction of the palmar aponeurosis, several authors have suggested that the basis of the condition should instead be placed in the palmar tissues superficial to the aponeurosis (Goyrand, 1833, and others). From histological studies MacCallum and Hueston (1962) concluded that, although the palmar aponeurosis is intimately involved in Dupuytren's contracture, this represents only one aspect of a change which may occur in any of the palmar connective tissues and is usually secondary to changes arising within the fibrofatty tissue on its superficial aspect.

In 1948 the author suggested that the strain to which

Figure 19.3

A, contracture of 14 years' standing in the case of a 69-year-old joiner. B, the retracted muscular bands at the level of the 3rd (ring) finger and of the little finger have been divided, and the normal character of the transverse palmar ligaments can be seen. C, the forceps indicate the thick retracted interdigital commisural ligament which is preventing the separation of the third and little fingers.

certain elements of the aponeurosis are subjected is essential in the pathogenesis of Dupuytren's contracture and that the disease originates in fibrillar ruptures within the aponeurosis (Skoog). This view was well supported in an experimental study by Larsen, Takagishi, and Posch (1960), who were able to reproduce the characteristic tissue changes in monkeys by traction causing fibre ruptures of the palmar aponeurosis. The observation reported here and first mentioned in 1963 (Skoog), that the transverse palmar ligament never becomes the site of pathological changes in Dupuytren's contracture, may be regarded as additional clinical evidence. It should then be pointed out that in no function of the hand are the fibres of this transverse band subject to tension or strain such as could reasonably be thought to cause them to rupture.

This conception of the pathogenesis of Dupuytren's contracture, formed on the basis of reported observations, leads to the practical conclusion that the transverse palmar ligament should be left alone in the surgical treatment of the diseased aponeurosis. The experience of such selective aponeurosectomy has been entirely satisfactory as will be reported later in this paper; no sign of recurrence has appeared at that site and the function of a well defined structure of the aponeurosis has been preserved.

Contrary to the transverse palmar ligament, the interdigital ligaments are in several functions of the hand subjected to strain: separation of the fingers will cause tension and these ligaments are also partly responsible for limitation of flexion of a finger when the other fingers are extended. The striking difference between the transverse interdigital ligaments and the transverse palmar ligament, in the respect that pathological changes occur only in the more distal of the two, can hardly be explained without the acceptance of strain as a causative factor. These morphological findings are thus of particular interest for our understanding of the nature and cause of the structural changes in Dupuytren's contracture; and they are obviously incompatible with most theories on the aetiology of this disease put forward through the years.

It should be emphasized that the pathogenesis and the aetiology of Dupuytren's contracture must be considered separately, as in any other disease. Several previously reported observations indicate that certain biomechanical qualities of the connective tissue in general, demonstrated in brittleness and decreased elasticity of the fibrous elements, are essential in creating a predispositions for the condition. The conception of the pathogenesis advanced here does not imply that the nature of the aponeurotic tissue differs from other fibrous elements of the individual concerned. The reason that the disease manifests itself in such a typical manner in the hand is readily explained as a consequence of the functional anatomy of the palmar aponeurosis

(Skoog, 1963). The pathological process itself is based on the fundamental principle of scar formation and contracture.

SURGICAL TREATMENT

PALMAR APONEUROSIS

In the past 15 years, 807 hands (621 patients) have been operated upon for Dupuytren's contracture in our Department. The numerous observations made on this material justify several conclusions of general interest; in this paper the comparisons are mainly limited to the quality of the results and the surgical techniques used in removing the palmar aponeurosis.

In the early part of my series, exposure was obtained according to the McIndoe (1946) method, through a wide incision in the distal palmar crease supplemented by separate Z-incisions on the fingers involved. The palmar aponeurosis was always radically excised, including the paratendinous septa down to their deep attachments. The subcutaneous and subaponeurotic fatty tissue, including the fat pads of the metacarpophalangeal region, were also extensively removed and thus the subaponeurotic anatomy became exposed in great detail. Following such extensive dissection, wound healing required about three weeks. Some of the patients subjected to this treatment have now been observed for more than 15 years. None of them has mentioned symptoms which could imply that the palmar aponeurosis is essential for the function of the hand. Several patients, however, complain of paraesthesia and pain in gripping, a feeling of the palm being 'unprotected', or that they have lost some strength in heavy gripping. On examination the palmar surface appears unnaturally flat, the normal palmar creases become less distinct, and a new pattern of finer creases has developed (Fig. 19.4). The fingers are easily hyperextended and the transverse palmar arch can be passively reversed. In some instances the pulsation of palmar arteries could be seen through the thin skin.

For the last five years our surgical approach in Dupuytren's contracture has been more conservative, leaving the surrounding delicate system of connective and fatty tissues as far as possible in place. It has also become a standard procedure to perform *selective aponeurosectomy*, i.e. to separate and preserve intact the transverse palmar ligament as well as the underlying paratendinous septa (Fig. 19.1E). In doing so these structures act as a safeguard in protecting the delicate anatomy of the deep palmar space during dissection. The neurovascular bundles are no longer isolated throughout their course; their freeing is mainly restricted to finger bases and adjacent parts of the palm, where the close relationship of the nerves and arteries to contracted bands may make such exposure useful for their protection. After com-

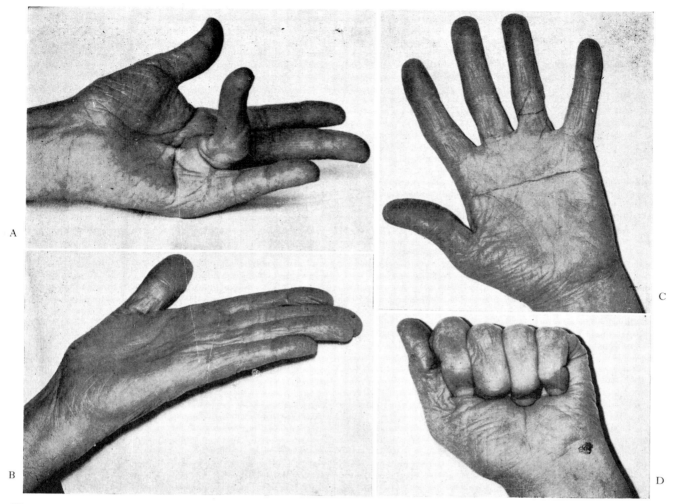

Figure 19.4
Although the retraction in this case is confined to the third finger (A), a radical fasciectomy has been carried out using a transverse palmar incision. Skin closure has been promoted by a Z-plasty at the level of the third (ring) finger. Thirteen years later (B, C, D), at the age of 77 years, the patient displays full finger extension and complete freedom in the palm of the hand.

pletion of the dissection an operative field is left in which the nerves, vessels, and muscles are veiled by sheets of fine connective tissue. The structures of the subaponeurotic space can therefore only to some extent be identified due to these sheets and surrounding fatty tissue. Another technical advantage in leaving the transverse palmar ligament is that, in closing the basic line of incision in the distal palmar crease, a few mattress sutures can be used for fixing the skin edges to the band, thus obliterating the palmar wound pocket (Fig. 19.5).

After limited excision of the palmar aponeurosis had been carried out as described, recovery was much quicker than following more radical procedures. Wound healing occurred in 10 to 12 days, and postoperative swelling of the fingers was markedly reduced. In hands in which the transverse fascial system of the palm was preserved in aponeurosectomy, there has been no recurrence within the palmar field of operation during the five years in which the method has been in use. When postoperative swelling and stiffness had subsided and sensation fully returned, the patients considered their hands to be normal in every respect. The configuration of the palm was normal with distinct transverse palmar creases, the metacarpophalangeal fat pads maintained, and the palmar arch preserved (Fig. 6). One patient in this group, who had previously undergone radical aponeurosectomy of his other hand, reported the strength and general feeling of that hand to be slightly, but definitely, inferior compared to the normal condition of the hand operated upon according to the more conservative technique.

Atraumatic surgical technique in the sense that the

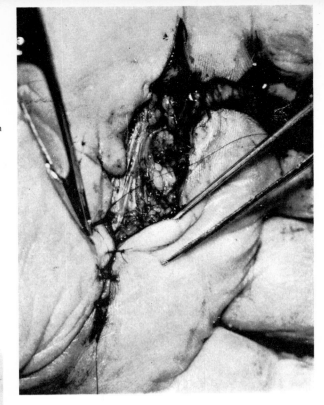

Figure 19.5
The skin suture has been secured to the transverse palmar ligament in such a way as to conceal the subcutaneous separation.

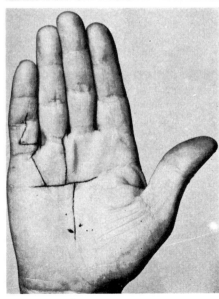

Figure 19.6
A, a contracture of 15 years' standing in a 55-year-old factory worker. B, C, D, the transverse palmar ligament has been left intact and the normal configuration of the palm can be seen; Note the transverse palmar flexion crease and the metacarpophalangeal fatty pads. The scars show that a Z-plasty has been carried out on the 5th finger.

A

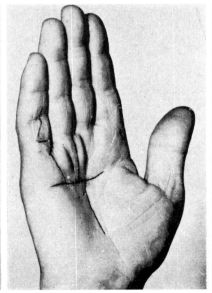

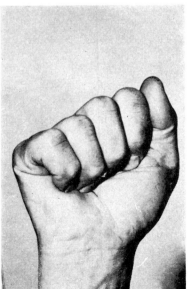

B   C   D

dissection is restricted to the palmar aponeurosis and its extensions has proved essential; surgical intervention outside the fascial system will unfavorably interfere with the lympathatic system of the hand and the venous return, both in the early postoperative period and later owing to the formation of scar tissue. Excessive scarring laid down in the process of repair may also cause recurrence of unpredictable nature, not necessarily related to the site of the palmar aponeurosis. Preservation of the subcutaneous fibrofatty tissues of the palm, particularly the metacarpophalangeal fat pads, also seems advantageous for protection and for moulding the surface of the hand in gripping. Apparently recurrences do not occur within these tissues, and reasonably so because the fibrous elements of the subcutaneous tissue layer are left loose when their deep attachments are cut in removing the aponeurosis.

Whether removal of aponeurotic tissue as a prophylactic measure should include pretendinous bands of normal appearance has to be decided upon in each individual case, considering the patient's age, disposition to the disease, etc. From a surgical and functional point of view, it makes little difference if the longitudinal bands are totally or only partially removed from the palm. One technical consideration should, however, be emphasized in this connection. From a prophylactic point of view it is recommended that in partial removal of the aponeurosis the line of resection is placed along the longitudinal fibres and care taken not to damage the bordering fibres of the portion left in place; the healing process of severed longitudinal fibres is likely to cause reappearance of the disease at that site.

It should be mentioned that this change in surgical technique for the removal of the palmar aponeurosis has been developed simultaneously with the introduction of a variety of skin incisions for exposure. Though this might to some extent be responsible for quicker wound healing, it is felt strongly that the new principle adopted for the dissection and resection of the aponeurosis has been decisive for the improvement of operative results.

SKIN AND SUBCUTANEOUS TISSUE

Suitable skin incisions in the surgical correction of contracted hands will be discussed briefly in this paper, and only with regard to the method for selected aponeurosectomy recommended.

The principle of restricting the removal of the aponeurosis to its longitudinal portions including diseased parts of the interdigital ligaments and as far as possible avoiding interference with fatty tissues and adjacent systems of thin connective tissue sheets makes good exposure essential. At the same time the limitation in dissection minimizes the need for exposure by wide undermining of palmar skin (Fig. 19.7). It has therefore been considered worth while to add still another pattern

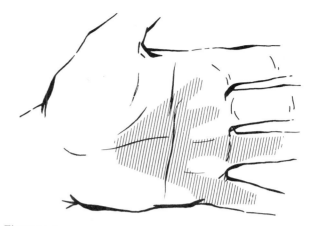

Figure 19.7
Diagram showing the extent of subcutaneous palmar separation required in carrying out a selective fasciectomy as described in the text, when the 4th and 5th longitudinal bands are affected.

of incisions to the numerous ones recommended for the surgical approach in Dupuytren's contracture (Fig. 19.6B). The basic line of incision is placed in the distal palmar crease, in length corresponding to the section of the aponeurosis to be removed. Distally extensions are made over present cords and carried on to the fingers, bifurcated contracted bands being exposed by Y-shaped incisions (Fig. 19.3C). Proximally a crease in the centre of the palm is incised, extending from the transverse incision line; the triangular skin flaps thus formed proximally are raised no further than to expose the border of the aponeurosis on either or both sides. Despite the extensiveness of these incisions, healing conditions have been excellent because of the good blood supply maintained due to limited undermining of the skin.

On the fingers the Z-plasty, introduced by McIndoe, still offers the best solution for wide exposure and for elongation of the shortened skin. Occasionally this ingenious procedure may be indicated to correct contracture in the distal portion of the palm (Fig. 19.8).

In areas where the pathological process has invaded the subcutaneous and dermal layers causing pits, deep furrows, and ridges, the palmar skin will regain most of its original surface when dissected off the underlying mass. Even when the skin has to be cut very thin in this manoeuvre its blood supply has proved to be sufficient, and after healing the skin has gradually become soft and pliable, indicating that the skin symptoms are only secondary and maintained by the mechanical effect of underlying contracted fibrous elements.

In no case have I found it necessary in primary treatment to replace palmar skin with skin grafts. Like Hueston (1963), I find the principal use of skin grafts to be after digital dissection of recurrent Dupuytren's contracture where the skin generally has decreased

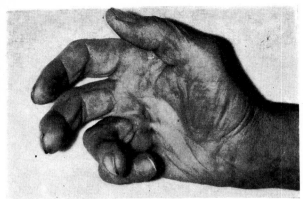

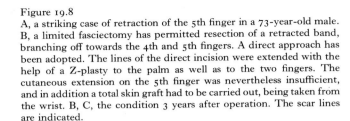

Figure 19.8
A, a striking case of retraction of the 5th finger in a 73-year-old male. B, a limited fasciectomy has permitted resection of a retracted band, branching off towards the 4th and 5th fingers. A direct approach has been adopted. The lines of the direct incision were extended with the help of a Z-plasty to the palm as well as to the two fingers. The cutaneous extension on the 5th finger was nevertheless insufficient, and in addition a total skin graft had to be carried out, being taken from the wrist. B, C, the condition 3 years after operation. The scar lines are indicated.

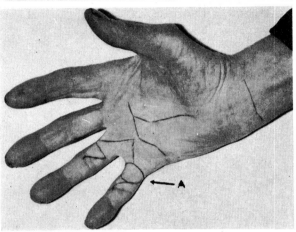

A

B

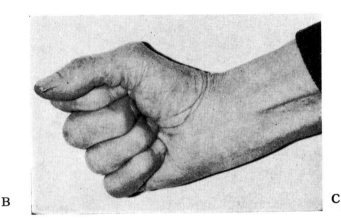

C

viability and elasticity, which makes it unfit for further rearrangement. Only in the case of a severely flexed finger of long standing may additional skin be needed at a primary operation to compensate for apparent shortage on the volar aspect (Fig. 19.8). The wrist then has been our first choice as a donor site for a fullthickness skin graft.

SUMMARY

Some original observations on the anatomy and pathology of the transverse elements of the palmar aponeurosis are reported. The transverse palmar ligament forms a continuous band, strictly limited to the midpalmar region with deep attachments at each end merging with the paratendinous septa bordering the compartment on the radial and the ulnar sides. Throughout its length the transverse band is intimately related to the underlying paratendinous septa and together they form a well defined fibrous tunnel system. The function of this separate anatomical structure is discussed, and related to observations on hands following its removal. In all stages of Dupuytren's contracture it was noticed that the transverse palmar band was not involved in the pathological process, this being confirmed as a constant feature in more than 300 consecutively operated hands. In marked contrast, the transverse fibres of the interdigital ligaments were frequently the site of pathological changes, resulting in contracted bands.

The striking lack of pathological changes in the transverse palmar ligament and their presence in the interdigital ligaments are obviously incompatible with most theories proposed on the aetiology of Dupuytren's contracture. Considering the anatomy of these bands, the difference in functional strain on their fibrous structures offers, however, a reasonable explanation. The observations made are regarded as additional clinical evidence in support of the author's previously expressed view, that Dupuytren's contracture develops as the result of ruptures of fibrils in the aponeurosis, affecting individuals with a general predisposition in their connective tissue. The pathological process itself is based on the fundamental principle of scar formation and contracture.

In the surgical treatment of Dupuytren's contracture *selective aponeurosectomy* is recommended, i.e., the transverse palmar ligament is separated from the contracted tissue and left intact together with the para-tendinous septa. In doing so the function of this fibrous tunnel system has been preserved; no recurrences were noticed at this site; healing time was reduced compared to that required following more radical procedures; and the functional restoration of the hand was also quicker. The principles for exposure of the contracted palmar aponeurosis are briefly discussed and a pattern of incisions is suggested to facilitate the dissection and to reduce the need for undermining of the skin.

REFERENCES

DUPUYTREN, G. (1832). *Leçons orales de clinique chirurgical,* vol. 1. Paris: Baillière.

GOYRAND, G. (1833). Nouvelles recherches sur la rétraction permanente des doigts. *Mémoires de l'Academie royal de Medicine,* **3,** 489.

HUESTON, J. T. (1963). *Dupuytren's Contracture.* Edinburgh: Livingstone.

KAPLAN, E. B. (1965). *Functional and Surgical Anatomy of the Hand.* Philadelphia: Lippincott.

LARSEN, R. D., TAKAGISHI, N. & POSCH, J. L. (1960). The pathogenesis of Dupuytren's contracture. *Journal of Bone and Joint Surgery,* **42A,** 993.

MACCALLUM, P. & HUESTON, J. T. (1962). The pathology of Dupuytren's contracture. *Australian and New Zealand Journal of Surgery,* **31,** 241.

McINDOE, A. (1946). Personal communication.

SKOOG, T. (1948). Dupuytren's contraction. *Acta chirurgica scandinavica,* Suppl. 139.

SKOOG, T. (1963). The pathogenesis and atiology of Dupuytren's contracture. *Plastic and Reconstructive Surgery,* **31,** 258.

20. SKIN REPLACEMENT IN DUPUYTREN'S CONTRACTURE

John T. Hueston

In discussing prognosis as a guide to the timing and extent of surgery in Dupuytren's contracture (Hueston, 1967) it was pointed out that 'radical local excision' *of both fascia and skin* with full thickness (Wolfe) graft replacement is often advised in young patients with a strong diathesis. That is, when recurrence has occurred after previous surgery, or where, by the rate of progress, and the presence of predisposing factors—such as epilepsy or alcoholism, a strong family history and ectopic deposits—it is considered likely that local recurrence will occur. It should be stressed again that the main indication for skin replacement in Dupuytren's contracture is to apply the important observation: *skin replacement prevents recurrence* (Fig. 20.1).

of interphalangeal joint stiffness. The role of the thigh flaps in the desperate salvage of digits with severe Dupuytren's contracture has been demonstrated by Clarkson (1966).

There are in general four circumstances in which skin replacement may need to be considered in Dupuytren's contracture:

(a) A skin defect from *correction of flexion deformity*; most frequently seen at the base of a digit where, despite transposition of Z-flaps there is still some longitudinal skin shortage (Fig. 20.2).

(b) *Devitalized skin*; if this is recognized at operation, free graft replacement using a whole thickness (Wolfe) graft is possible. If this skin necrosis is not detected

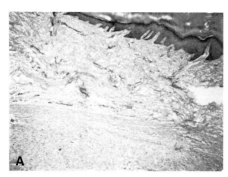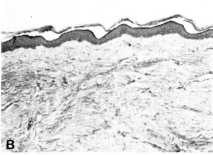

Figure 20.1
Photomicrograph of palmar skin and subcutaneous tissue immediately beneath the dermis. A, recurrent digital nodule of Dupuytren's contracture. B, Beneath a full thickness graft of 4 years' standing there is only scar tissue and no evidence of recurrence of the hyperplastic Dupuytren's tissue.

Whenever the possibility arises that skin replacement may be needed after fasciectomy, more than the usual care should be taken to retain the fibrous sheath of the flexor tendons, to allow the direct application of a free graft. Should the flexor tendons become exposed, the problem of skin cover would become immensely more complex, perhaps even requiring flap transfers from the other arm or the medial thigh.

The writer considers that cross-finger flaps are better avoided in young patients with Dupuytren's contracture because not only is it possible that the donor finger will itself develop Dupuytren's contracture later and require a volar dissection, but new deposits of Dupuytren's contracture could be initiated in the donor finger by such interference.

However in an elderly patient, with less risk of recurrence, a cross-finger flap may be considered, although this would introduce the additional hazard

early, then a free graft applied after removal of the skin slough will need to be a split thickness graft and the result will be correspondingly inferior.

(c) In *recurrent Dupuytren's contracture* the overlying skin may be so densely infiltrated and fixed to the new deforming tissue that an adequate dissection must render this skin ischaemic. If the circulation is preserved, the skin must be still too heavily infiltrated with Dupuytren's tissue to be reasonably left in the area. This dilemma arises most often when recurrence has occurred more than once. After having been forced to use full thickness (Wolfe) grafts in such circumstances it was subsequently found that, although further deposits of Dupuytren's contracture occurred in adjacent areas, none appeared beneath the free skin grafts (Fig. 20.1). It thus appears that *the removal of the volar skin of the palm or digit removes with it the mechanism responsible for the production of recurrent Dupuytren's contracture.*

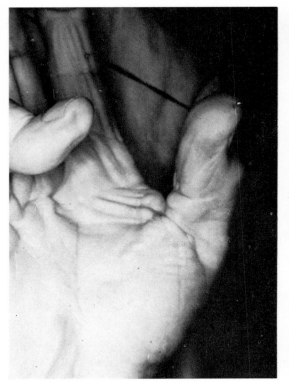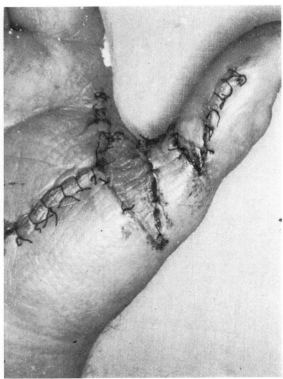

Figure 20.2
A combination of local flap and complementary full thickness free graft at the level of the base of the thumb.

Berger (1892) and Lexer (1931) advocated radical skin excision in Dupuytren's contracture on the analogy with burn scar contraction, but the phenomenon of freedom from recurrence beneath the grafts, reported by Piulachs and Mir y Mir (1952), Gordon (1957 and 1964) and Hueston (1962) has stimulated the reintroduction of free graft replacement of the skin in recurrent Dupuytren's contracture.

(d) *Prophylactic skin excision to prevent recurrence* in a patient with a strong diathesis to the production of Dupuytren's tissue, would seem at first to be an extremely radical step. Tubiana (1963) wisely advised that 'it is generally agreed that skin excision for dermal infiltration is a sacrifice that is not necessary, because these infiltrated areas regain much of their elasticity postoperatively; very few surgeons advocate systematic dermal excision on a prophylactic basis'. However, in those young patients with a strong diathesis as judged from an early age of onset, a diffuse disease with rapid progress, dermal fixation and usually with ectopic deposits, the likelihood of later surgery for recurrence is so great—and this later surgery is likely to be so much more difficult, involving dissection of neurovascular bundles and fibrous flexor sheath from the new tissue mass—that, in such highly selected cases, a pro-phylactic skin excision and Wolfe graft replacement is performed.

The digit is first dissected through a longitudinal incision (Fig. 20.3A); no digital skin is sacrificed until it is certain that the entire flexor sheath has been preserved intact (Fig. 20.3B), and therefore capable of providing a perfect bed for the free graft. Then the flaps are widely excised (Fig. 20.3C) and, with appropriated darts at interphalangeal joint levels, a full thickness (Wolfe) graft is sutured into place (Fig. 20.3D).

Healing takes less than two weeks and movements are commenced at about the same time as after any other form of skin closure. In these young patients good joint movements are preserved (Fig. 20.4), and recurrence prevented.

The need arises in exceptional cases to return to Lexer's method of radical skin replacement (Fig. 20.5).

There is probably great aetiological significance in this observation that the behaviour of the palmar and digital volar tissues in patients with Dupuytren's contracture is altered when the overlying skin has been changed. It emphasizes our still great ignorance of the physiology, and hence of the pathology, of this connective tissue compartment enclosed between the palmar aponeurosis and the skin of the palm.

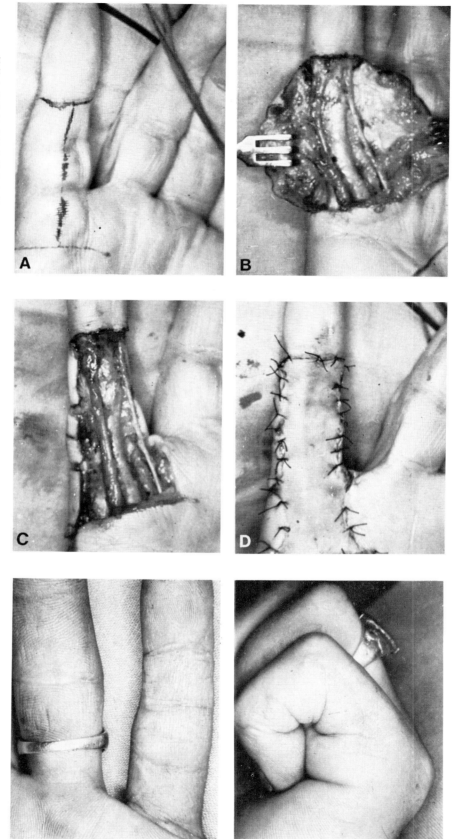

Figure 20.3
Primary full thickness resurfacing of the little finger in a young patient with aggressive Dupuytren's contracture where poor prognosis is anticipated (A, B). The finger is exposed by a longitudinal incision and both skin and fascia resected, carefully preserving the flexor sheath. C, after excision of fascia and skin, darts are made at the interphalangeal joint levels. D, resurfacing of the finger by a full-thickness graft taken from the inner aspect of the same arm.

Figure 20.4
Four years after total resurfacing of the volar aspect of the left little finger by a full thickness skin graft in a 28-year-old male with a poor prognosis assessed on general and local grounds. No recurrence is present and full movements are seen (reproduced by permission of the Editor, *British Journal of Plastic Surgery*).

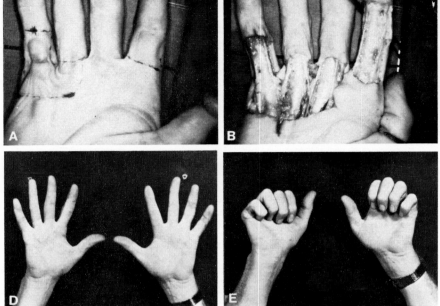

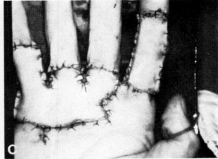

Figure 20.5
A, recurrent Dupuytren's contracture on little finger and distal palm 2 years after two fasciectomies. Extensive dermal invasion in primary lesions on index and base of middle fingers. B, C, skin has been excised along with the fascia from the volar aspect of the index finger and proximal half of the little finger and the distal part of the palm related to middle, ring and little fingers. Full thickness skin graft replacement from the inner aspect of the same arm, the donor site having been split skin grafted. D, E, two years later there is no evidence of local recurrence or limitation of movement.

REFERENCES

BERGER, P. (1892). Traitment de la rétraction de l' aponeurose palmaire par une autoplastie. *Bulletin de l' Académie de Médecine,* Paris, **56,** 608.

CLARKSON, P. (1966). *Clinical Surgery,* p. 229. London: Butterworths.

GORDON, S. (1957). Dupuytren's contracture, recurrence and extension following surgical treatment. *British Journal of Plastic Surgery,* **9,** 286.

GORDON, S. (1964a). Dupuytren's contracture, plantar involvement. *British Journal of Plastic Surgery,* **17,** 421.

GORDON, S. (1964b). Dupuytren's contracture, the use of free skin grafts in treatment. *Transactions of the International Congress of Plastic Surgeons, Washington,* **963.**

HUESTON, J. T. (1962). Digital Wolfe grafts in recurrent Dupuytren's contracture. *Plastic and Reconstructive Surgery,* **29,** 342.

HUESTON, J. T. (1963). Recurrent Dupuytren's contracture. *Plastic and Reconstructive Surgery,* **31,** 66.

HUESTON, J. T. (1963). *Dupuytren's Contracture.* Edinburgh: Livingstone.

HUESTON, J. T. (1965a). Dupuytren's contracture, the trend to conservatism. *Annals of the Royal College of Surgeons of England,* **36,** 134.

HUESTON, J. T. (1965b). The skin in Dupuytren's contracture. In *Studies in Pathology,* p. 151. Melbourne University Press.

HUESTON, J. T. (1967). Prognosis as a guide to the timing and extent of surgery in Dupuytren's contracture. In *Maladie de Dupuytren,* p. 69. Paris: Expansion Scientifique Française.

LEXER, E. (1931). *Die gesamte Wiederherstillungschirgie,* 2nd edn, vol. 2. Leipzig:

PIULACHS, P. & MIR y MIR, L. (1952). Consideraciones sobre la enfermedad de Dupuytren. *Folia Clinica internacional (Barcelona),* **2,** 8.

TUBIANA, R. (1963). Les temps cutanés dans la traitment chirurgical de la maladie de Dupuytren. *Annales de chirurgie plastique,* **8,** 157.

21. OPEN FASCIOTOMY AND FULL THICKNESS SKIN GRAFT IN THE CORRECTION OF DIGITAL FLEXION DEFORMITY

Richard I. Gonzalez

Postoperative morbidity following the surgical treatment of Dupuytren's contracture as manifested by delayed healing, joint stiffness, and pain is well known. As Howard (1959) has stated, 'The only major problem in the surgical treatment of Dupuytren's contracture is the prevention of postoperative stiffness of the small finger joints.' And as Shaw and Barclay (1957) noted, 'The overriding consideration leading to a successful (surgical) result is to restore a healed hand to normal use within three months of operation.' The degree of postoperative morbidity, in my experience, has been almost proportionate to the extent of the surgical procedure, the more extensive the procedure, the greater the morbidity. The simplest surgical procedure, subcutaneous fasciectomy, carries very little morbidity yet in my experience, in progressive disease, provides only temporary relief of the contracture. However, radical palmar fasciectomy with or without finger dissections, though carrying a high degree of postoperative morbidity, does not guarantee prevention of recurrence of the disease. In 1951 Hamlin recognized this seeming enigma and advocated limited palmar fasciectomy in the hope of reducing postoperative morbidity. He recommended excision of the diseased fascia alone and was able to return his patients to 'usual occupation' 12 to 30 days postoperatively in contra-indication to the average 118 days needed following the classical radical fasciectomy.

In this report there was, however, no indication as to the extent of finger contractures v. localized palmar involvement. In 1961 Hueston reported on a larger series of patients utilizing local fasciectomy plus multiple Z-plasties to lengthen the secondarily shortened volar skin over the contracted fingers. Of these patients 12·5 per cent recovered full flexion within three weeks, and 84·5 per cent in six weeks following surgery. In neither series was recurrence a major problem. In the hope of further reducing postoperative morbidity and approaching the ideal of full return of function within three weeks following surgery I substituted inset full thickness skin grafts for Z-plasties to overcome volar finger skin shortness. By transecting the contracting fascial band and skin at its point of maximal tension and inserting full thickness skin grafts into the defect, dissection and undermining is kept to a minimum and healing and return of function is rapid. The use of full thickness skin grafts as an adjunct

TABLE 1   Operative experience in 100 contracted joints

Patients	39
Male	30
Female	9
Age range	18–91
Average age	58·6
Past history	
Arthritis	19
Bursitis	12
Heart 'trouble'	5
Family history of Dupuytren's contracture	12
Maternal	6
Paternal	6
Previous treatment	
Surgery	17
X-ray	1
Cortisone	1
Ultra sound	1
Distribution of disease	
Palm	31
Thumb	6
Index	4
Long	12
Ring	17
Little	34
Contracted joints	
Proximal joint	46
Average lack of extension	$-46°$
Middle joint	44
Average lack of extension	$-49°$
Distal joint	10
Average lack of extension	$-33°$
Total operations	46
Type operation	
Limited palmar fasciectomy + full thickness skin grafts (finger)	31
Full thickness skin grafts only (finger)	15
Donor sites	
Groin	48
Foot	12
Ante cubital fossa	3
Total free full thickness skin grafts	63

* This series demonstrates the usual sex and age distribution as well as the association of Dupuytren's contracture with other forms of coexisting collagen disease. The high incidence of previous surgical treatment indicates the applicability of this technique to recurrent or progressive Dupuytren's contracture. The low incidence of palmar involvement is a reflection of the fact that no cases of palmar involvement without finger joint contractures were included in this series.

to the treatment of Dupuytren's contracture is not new. Gordon (1948), Skoog (1967) and Hueston (1969) have all recommended the use of Wolfe grafts for replacement of avascular palmar skin. However, no one to my knowledge has used them as insets or additions to lengthen shortened skin. I have released 100 contracted finger joints in this manner over the past 11 years, 84 per cent have recovered full flexion and extension within 21 days following surgery and to date there have been no recurrences of the contractures.

TECHNIQUE

Under either general or local anaesthesia, the point of maximal tension of the contracting band is marked and a transverse skin incision is made to each mid-lateral line. The neurovascular bundles are identified and mobilized by spreading longitudinally with sharp pointed scissors. After the bundles are well visualized, all fascial bands are totally divided transversely, usually allowing the finger to extend completely (Fig. 21.1). Shortened volar joint capsules may restrict full extension but are best mobilized postoperatively by the use of a dorsal clock spring splint and not by capsulotomy. The proximal palmar remnant of the fascial band can be excised through short vertical or transverse incisions (Fig. 21.2). This can be eliminated without jeopardizing the end result, as remnants of the released fascial bands soften and largely disappear. The site of operation is then changed to the donor site, either the groin or instep of the foot. Foot skin most resembles finger skin in texture, colour and thickness; however, the size of a

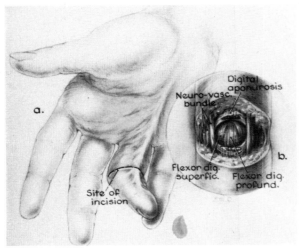
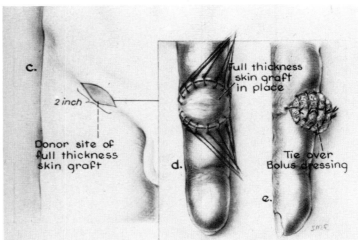

Figure 21.1
Operative technique (reproduced by permission of the Editor, *Clinical Orthopedics*).

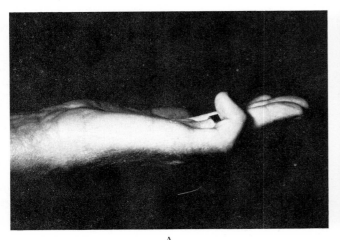
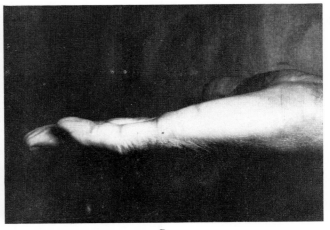

A   B

Figure 21.2
A, severe flexion deformity of the left little finger principally at the interphalangeal joint level. B, almost complete correction after full thickness skin graft at the level of the middle phalanx.

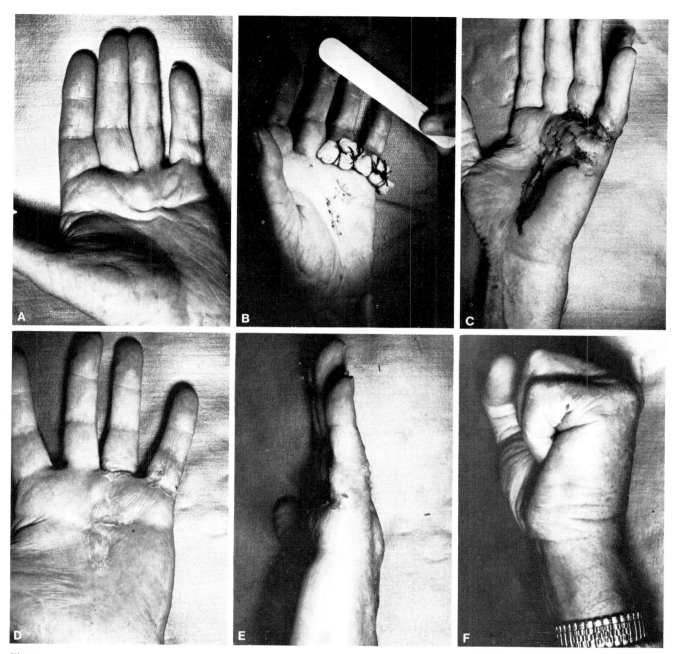

Figure 21.3
A, moderately severe flexion deformity of the metacarpophalangeal joint of the ring and little finger. B, partial palmar fasciectomy and full thickness skin graft at the level of the incision at the base of each finger. C, one week postoperatively on removal of primary dressings. D, E, F, sound healing and good movements obtained by the 20th day.

graft that can be taken from the instep is limited unless one is willing to split graft the donor site. Another disadvantage of using the foot as a donor site is the necessity to restrict weight bearing until healing is complete. The groin as a donor site provides a source for large grafts and it has the advantage of ease of closure. The disadvantage is that of hyperpigmentation of the graft, particularly in dark-skinned patients. If one leaves a thin layer of dermis in the base of the donor site, closure is greatly facilitated and undermining is not necessary. Quite large donor areas can be closed with a simple running suture. Care should be taken to remove the graft from the lateral aspect of the groin where there are few hair follicles. The free graft is carefully sutured into the denuded area of the finger. Sutures are placed 2 to 3 millimetres apart, left long and tied over the bolus of wet cotton (Fig. 21.1E). Postoperative bleeding, haematoma formation or 'graft take' have not been a problem; however, if a graft is lost an immediate cross finger flap would be necessary to protect the exposed flexor tendons. A volar plaster splint is incorporated in the dressing, to keep the grafted finger at rest. The bolus is removed at 7 days and skin sutures at 10 days.

Supervised active exercises are carried out until full flexion and extension is achieved. In order to achieve maximal flexor power to the small finger joints, each finger joint should be stabilized by the patient by firmly holding the finger just proximal to each joint and vigorously contracting the flexor musculature. Only by such vigorous exercise can early return of full flexion be achieved. It is the surgeon's responsibility to make certain that these exercises are carried out continuously and properly.

DISCUSSION

Most grafts healed well within 10 days following surgery (Figs. 21.2, 21.3). In a few there was delay in healing of the superficial layers of the graft. This did not interfere with the institution of vigorous active exercises. In a large number (13) of the cases full flexion was achieved immediately after the bolus and sutures had been removed from the grafts (10 days) but 98 per cent had recovered full flexion within 40 days. One full thickness skin graft was lost due to haemorrhage and secondary infection. This was in an alcoholic woman who fell three days postoperatively on her hand fracturing her splint. She failed to return for postoperative visits. In this case both tendons and neurovascular bundle sloughed. If a cross finger flap had been placed on the exposed tendons I am sure the function of the finger could have been preserved. One other patient failed to recover full flexion and extension of his finger. This was a 91-year-old gentleman whose little finger had been firmly flexed into his palm for 25 years. The

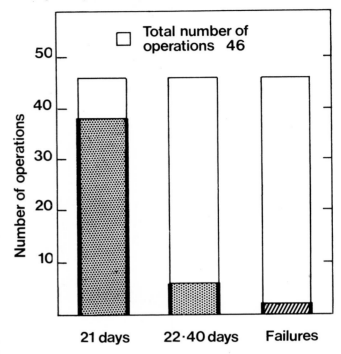

TABLE 3   Delay in recovery of full flexion

TABLE 2

Operative results	
Postoperative morbidity: (Chart 1)	
Recovery full flexion 21 days postoperative	38 (83 per cent)
Recovery full flexion 40 days postoperative	44 (96 per cent)
Recurrence	0
Progression	0
Follow up: Average (Chart 2)	3.5 years
Range	1.5 to 11.5 years
Complications	
Nerve damage	0
Haematoma	0
Infection with loss of graft	1

middle joint failed to respond to postoperative splinting. Though extension was improved the patient did not recover full flexion or extension postoperatively. These two failures illustrate two potential shortcomings of the technique. First when a graft is lost it is imperative to cover the exposed tendons and nerves with pedicle tissue and second in long-standing contractures in the very aged total recovery of flexion and extension should not be expected.

Full return of function was achieved within 21 days following surgery in 85 per cent of the cases in which finger contractures were present preoperatively. One hundred contracted joints were released with loss of only one graft and without recurrence of the disease. The total lack of recurrent contracture of released joints has been an unexpected dividend of this technique. One might theorize that in advanced Dupuytren's contracture the skin overlying the contracted fascial bands is diseased and has an intrinsic potential of contracture in itself and that by dividing the soft tissue and interposing normal skin this potential is eliminated. Hueston (1969, and personal communication) has theorized along similar lines, and feels that all the overlying abnormal skin should be replaced in potentially progressive or recurrent disease. I feel that the main value of this simplified technique, however, is that it offers simple surgical control of progressive and recurrent disease with minimal postoperative morbidity.

SUMMARY

Haematoma formation, delay in healing, pain, stiffened finger joints are frequent complications following classical surgical approaches to Dupuytren's contracture. The high degree of postoperative morbidity has discouraged many from recommending surgical treatment for this relatively benign condition. A new surgical approach to the disease that can correct the contractures without the attendant morbidity is urgently needed. By treating Dupuytren's as any other scar contracture (division of the contracting soft tissue at its point of maximal tension and interposing normal free full thickness skin) postoperative morbidity can be markedly decreased.

REFERENCES

GORDON, S. (1948). Dupuytren's contracture. *Canadian Medical Association Journal,* **58,** 543.

HAMLIN, E. (1952). Limited fasciectomy of Dupuytren's contracture. *Annals of Surgery,* **135,** 194.

HOWARD, L. D. (1959). Dupuytren's contracture: a guide for management. *Clinical Orthopaedics* No. 15, 118.

HUESTON, J. T. (1961). Limited Fasciectomy for Dupuytren's Contracture. *Plastic and Reconstructive Surgery,* **27,** 569.

HUESTON, J. T. (1969). Control of recurrent Dupuytren's contracture by skin replacement. *British Journal of Plastic Surgery,* **22,** 152.

HUESTON, J. T. Personal communication.

SHAW, M. H. & BARCLAY, T. L. (1957). Dupuytren's contracture—the results of radical fasciectomy. *Transactions of the International Society of Plastic Surgeons. First Congress* 1955, p. 428. Baltimore: Williams & Wilkins.

SKOOG, T. (1967). Dupuytren's contracture: pathogenesis and surgical treatment. *Surgical Clinics of North America,* **47,** 433.

ADDENDUM

Since submission of this paper for publication all cases have been followed for a minimum of three years. There has been one recurrent contracture of a previously released middle joint. The secondary contracture was easily corrected by division of the skin and subcutaneous band plus insert of a free full-thickness skin graft just distal to the previously placed grafts.

I do not believe that Dupuytren's contracture is 'curable' by surgical means. However, the disease can be controlled by this single surgical approach. As no deep scar is formed in this technique, secondary release, if needed, is a simple and safe procedure.

22. THE OPEN PALM TECHNIQUE IN DUPUYTREN'S CONTRACTURE

C. R. McCash

In 1832 Baron Dupuytren laid down the essential principles in the operative treatment of the disease which bears his name. These were as follows:

1. Transverse incisions in the skin creases.
2. Division of the fascial bands responsible for the contracture.
3. Splinting of the fingers in extension for four weeks after the operation.
4. Wounds left open and allowed to heal by granulation.

Looking back on this method in the light of present day knowledge, it is apparent that Dupuytren's results must have been adversely affected by the fact that he was only operating upon very advanced cases, and without anaesthesia, that he did not attempt to excise the diseased fascia, and that he may not have appreciated the importance of early active movements in maintaining the circulation in the hand. In spite of these handicaps his results were remarkably successful.

Today we have the advantages of the 'bloodless field', safe anaesthesia, antibiotics, and a much better understanding of wound healing and skin tension, and yet postoperative complications can still occur and cause a prolonged and painful convalescence.

In Dupuytren's contracture the shortening and puckering of the palm skin is often the first sign of the

disease and is evident long before invasion of the tendon sheaths has led to a flexion contracture. When such skin has been dissected up it is found to have lost its normal elasticity and its vitality is therefore impaired. If it is split up into flaps it is liable to develop areas of marginal necrosis especially if it is stretched by pressure from a haematoma, swollen with oedema, or pulled upon by active movements. Skin sloughs developing in this way are very susceptible to infection with its sequelae of pain, muscle spasm, finger oedema and joint stiffness.

In plastic surgery the generally recognized method of treating a flexion contracture due to scar contracture of the soft tissues over a major joint is to commence by carrying a thorough excision of the scarred skin and the contracted bands of deep fascia. When the joint can be fully extended without tension, the surgeon next proceeds to cover the skin defect with either a free graft or a flap. If the dissection has exposed bare tendon or bone a full thickness skin flap is preferred. The limb

Figure 22.1
A, B, 55-year-old male treated by the open palm method on both hands.

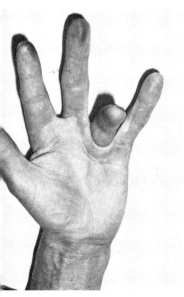
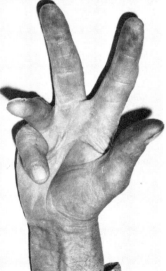
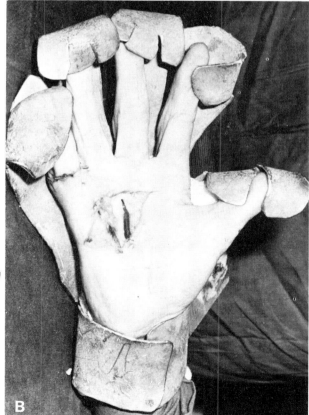

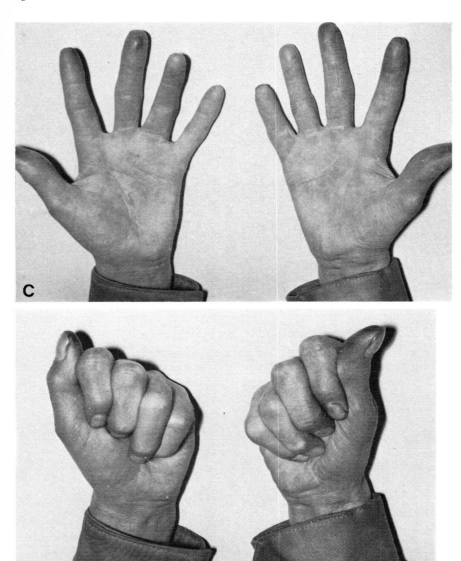

Figure 22.1
C, D, left hand 3 months
post-operatively; right hand 6
months post-operatively.

is then fixed with the joint extended for a long enough period to allow for sound healing before the commencement of active movements.

Now Dupuytren's disease is essentially a flexion contracture and one might expect a split skin graft to act equally well after a palmar fasciectomy. Unfortunately free grafts on the palm of the hand even of full thickness as advocated by Kanavel *et al.* (1929) are not as satisfactory as those applied to the flexor aspect of the knee or elbow. In the first place it is difficult in this situation to prevent serous effusion or haematoma and also in Dupuytren's the graft is sutured to skin which is already reduced in vitality by disease and the dissection. If the graft does not take 100 per cent the areas of necrosis readily become infected. Then again to give the graft sufficient time to consolidate means that hand movements must be restricted for longer than a week. This in turn slows down the blood and lymph circulation and increases the tendency to statis oedema. The other objection to a free graft in the palm is that it is not suitable where the dissection has exposed the flexor tendons by the removal of the tendon sheaths.

Recognizing these facts the surgeon has several alternative methods of repairing the skin shortage:
1. Plan the incisions to close with Z-plasties.
2. Transpose a flap from the dorsum.

3. When it is necessary to amputate a finger use its filleted skin as a flap.

4. Simply close the palm incision with the fingers flexed and trust that finger extension can be restored by exercises after the wound has healed.

Each of these techniques has its place in suitable cases and can give good results, but yet another, the 'open palm', can also give a high percentage of success with greater freedom from complications and less discomfort during convalescence.

PRINCIPLES OF THE OPEN PALM TECHNIQUE

1. By making the incisions as Dupuytren did in the transverse skin creases, each area of skin which is dissected up has a double blood supply and therefore is more resistant to infection and heals better.

2. By advancing the undermined skin bridge flaps proximally and distally with the fingers extended, the whole of the skin shortage is accepted by the main incision in the distal palmar crease which remains wide open. The other incisions close easily without tension and the central defect gives perfect drainage so that no haematoma can occur.

3. After a week's complete rest of the hand in a pressure dressing the patient must start to use the hand actively, and each night wear a splint which keeps the metacarpophalangeal joints extended.

4. By laying down a simple routine during convalescence the patient is able to treat himself at home without physiotherapy and the period of hospitalization is reduced to only a few days. All that is necessary is for him to attend the 'hand clinic' at weekly intervals.

OPERATIVE TECHNIQUE OF 'OPEN PALM'

Anaesthesia. General or brachial block.

Haemostasis. Pneumatic cuff and Esmarch bandage. After removal, bleeding arrested by pressure—no ligatures.

Incisions. Transverse in skin creases.

Dissection. Only the diseased fascia, recognized by its tension and lack of normal lustre, is removed. Distally the dissection is not carried further than the proximal interphalangeal joints. It has been found that to go further than this point at the primary operation is liable to hamper the full use of the hand during convalescence as well as increasing the danger of digital nerve damage. In most cases the patients are quite satisfied with the improvement in function they have gained, but in those who insist on a completely straight finger, the intricate dissection which is required can be carried out at a later date under 'digital block' anaesthesia.

Skin closure. With the fingers extended on the 'lead hand' splint the actual skin shortage is apparent and is often much more than one would expect. The proximal and distal incisions are then sutured.

The skin defect. The main incision in the distal palmar crease is now wide open with tendons and nerves exposed in its base. If its skin edges do not lie flatly and so leave spaces beneath, they are loosely tacked down with nylon mattress sutures.

The dressing. The tourniquet is released and after bleeding has stopped the open wound is covered with one layer of tuille gras and a pad of polyvinyl sponge. Over this a firm pressure dressing to the entire hand is applied with a volar plaster of Paris slab pressed well against the palm as it sets.

After-care. Arm elevated in a sling. No antibiotics unless there is pyrexia. Patient goes home on the third day to attend as an outpatient on the seventh day.

First dressing. One week after the operation the hand is taken down completely. The base of the open wound is now covered with a thin layer of granulations and the fingers can be moved actively without pain. A light non-adherent dressing is applied, sufficient to exclude dust infection but not to interfere with finger movements. The patient is instructed to use the hand for every light duty that he can do—writing, typing, piano playing, and very soon car driving. He is given a light spring wire splint to be applied over his dressing and worn at night only. The use of this can cease when the wounds are completely healed.

Subsequent dressings. These are at weekly intervals. The open wound which heals rapidly by marginal epithelialisation is soon reduced to a narrow fissure and finally closed in from two to five weeks.

DISCUSSION AND RESULTS

The 'open palm' technique is presented as yet another way of overcoming the skin shortage in the operation of palmar fasciectomy. It fulfills the original principles laid down by Baron Dupuytren, modified, however, by the advances in technique which orthopaedic and plastic surgeons have contributed to surgery of the hand.

This method is quite unsuitable for elderly patients with advanced secondary joint contractures and also in those who are unwilling or unable to co-operate in their own after-care.

The open wound appears to cause very little discomfort while it is healing and the necessity of wearing a light dressing over it is a small price to pay for the greater freedom from stiffness and muscle spasm.

In a series of 150 cases treated between 1959 and 1966, only a very few developed a mild local infection, which rapidly subsided with Furacin dressings. A serious discharge from the wound is normally seen and this may well account for the remarkable freedom from oedema which is a feature of convalescence.

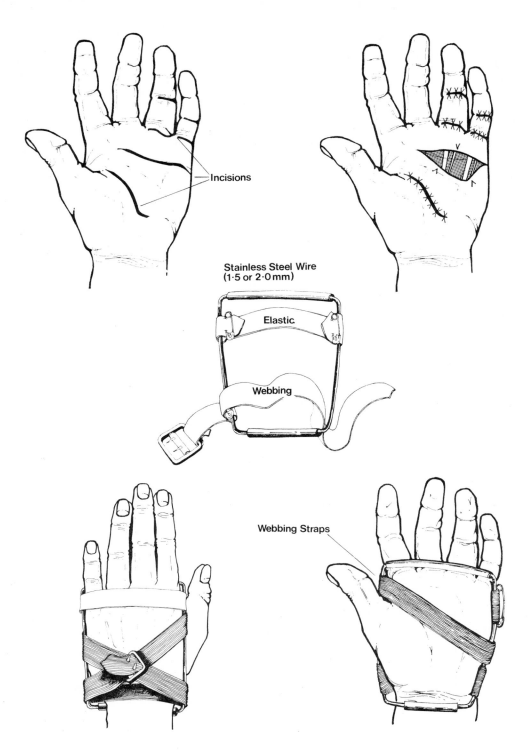

Incisions

Stainless Steel Wire
(1·5 or 2·0 mm)

Elastic

Webbing

Webbing Straps

Figure 22.3
Drawings showing details of the night splint.

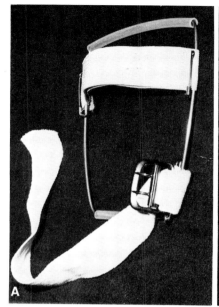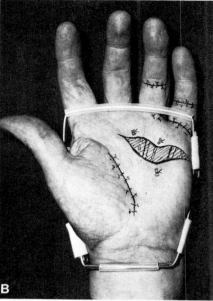

Figure 22.2
A, night splint made of strong wire with polythene covering to retain MP extension by elastic band across the back of the hand and the strap across the back of the wrist; B, such a night splint leaves the palm open for dressing and allows finger movement.

As regards disfigurement by scarring, this is only apparent in the early stages and by the end of a year or less is no more noticeable than after fasciectomy by other techniques.

It has also been suggested that the wound must close by circumferential contracture. It is to prevent this that I insist on the patient continuing to wear a night splint until the wound is healed and even if contracture does play a part in the healing process, it does not pull down the fingers, so is of no consequence.

SUMMARY

Some degree of skin contracture in the palm is present in probably 90 per cent of cases of Dupuytren's contracture. It is the flexion deformity of the metacarpophalangeal joints which causes the greatest disablement and the primary object of the fasciectomy should be to release them. Such release cannot be complete unless there is sufficient palm skin to permit of their full extension. This can only be ensured by the addition of either a full-thickness skin flap or by a free graft, or by natural regeneration of the skin as in the 'open palm' method. The 'open palm' wound has certain advantages over skin grafts. It acts as an open drain to the palm preventing haematoma in the early postoperative phase and oedema during the later stage when active movements commence. It affords complete relaxation of the palm skin in the 'extended' position and all the patient has to do is to restore the ability to flex his fingers. This he can do at home without physiotherapy, and therefore is made to feel he is contributing actively in the process of recovery.

23. *VOLAR CAPSULECTOMY OF THE PROXIMAL INTERPHALANGEAL JOINT IN DUPUYTREN'S CONTRACTURE*

Raymond M. Curtis

The surgeon who is called upon to treat the flexion contracture of the fingers, secondary to Dupuytren's contracture, frequently finds, after carrying out a thorough resection of the thickened fascia within the finger, that the finger still fails to fully extend at the proximal interphalangeal joint. Hueston reports uncorrectable deformity of the proximal interphalangeal joint as being present in 26 per cent of one hundred and twelve patients with interphalangeal joint flexion operated upon. He has suggested, in some instances, a separation of the oblique collateral ligament from the neck of the proximal phalanx as a method of improving this flexion contracture.

If the degree of flexion contracture is mild and one radically removes the thickened fascia in certain instances, with proper splinting postoperatively, one may achieve an improvement in the degree of extension. There are, however, patients in whom the contracture is so severe, and in whom no correction is obtained following fasciectomy, where the procedure of amputation of the finger may be entertained as a result of the inadequate correction. It is in this patient that an operative capsulectomy may salvage a useless finger.

MECHANICAL FACTORS LIMITING EXTENSION OF THE INTERPHALANGEAL JOINTS

The finger which has been flexed for a long period of time as a result of Dupuytren's contracture may lack complete extension for a number of anatomical reasons:

1. Inadequate skin over the volar surface of the finger.
2. Contraction of the fascia within the finger.
3. Contracture of the flexor tendon sheath within the finger.
4. Contracted flexor muscles or adherent flexor tendons.
5. Contracture of the volar plate of the capsular ligament.
6. Adherence of the retinacular ligament to the collateral ligaments or shortening of the retinacular ligament.
7. Adherence of the accessory volar ligament to the neck and condyle of the proximal phalanx.

OPERATIVE TECHNIQUE AND POSTOPERATIVE TREATMENT

The finger is approached through a mid-line incision and a complete fasciectomy is carried out, care being made to identify the volar digital nerves and arteries throughout the dissection. The skin incision is illustrated in Figs. 23.1, 23.2. This demonstrates the conversion of the straight line incision by the Z-plasty technique. Such a multiple Z gives additional length to the contracted skin over the flexor surface of the finger. When an adequate release of the flexion contracture is not obtained by the fascial excision, a section of the volar plate on either side of the flexor tendon is excised, as demonstrated in Fig. 23.5, together with a portion of the accessory volar ligament. As a rule, one may leave a small ribbon of volar plate over the central portion of the joint (Fig. 23.6). The operator tests the joint to see if easy extension can be obtained. If not, the retinacular ligaments should be tested; if they are tight and holding the finger into flexion, they should be sectioned on either side of the proximal interphalangeal joint (Fig. 23.3).

In a few instances the flexor profundus tendon has been standing, it may be necessary to excise the entire volar plate (Fig. 7), remove a portion of the flexor tendon sheath and section the contracted flexor sublimis tendon.

In a few instances the flexor profundus tendon has been lengthened in the forearm.

Light rubber band traction to the tip of the finger is started seventy-two hours after surgery by using a splint which holds the metacarpophalangeal joints in moderate flexion. The plaster splint extends dorsally from the forearm and hand, over the proximal phalanx, to a point just distal to the proximal interphalangeal joint. From the edge of this cast, just distal to the proximal interphalangeal joint, is attached an outrigger. This allows one to exert slight rubber band traction to the terminal phalanx of the finger in the early postoperative period in order that extension of the finger may be encouraged along with early flexion. The flexion at the metacarpophalangeal joint by the splint protects the palmar incision and prevents elevation of the palmar skin flaps during this early postoperative period.

It may be necessary to perform a volar capsulectomy of the metacarpophalangeal joint in order to achieve full extension of the finger.

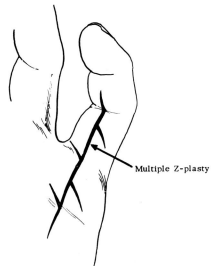

Multiple Z-plasty

Figure 23.1
Skin incision including plan of Z-plasty.

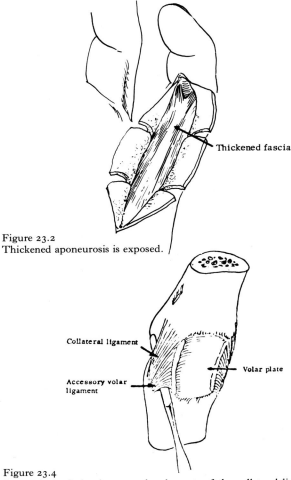

Thickened fascia

Figure 23.2
Thickened aponeurosis is exposed.

Collateral ligament

Accessory volar ligament

Volar plate

Figure 23.4
Anatomical relation between the elements of the collateral ligament main element, the accessory element and the volar plate of the joint at the level of the proximal interphalangeal joint. It can be seen that the lateral ligament and accessory ligament do not attach on the palmar aspect of the condyle of the proximal phalanx.

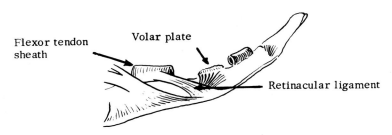

Flexor tendon sheath

Volar plate

Retinacular ligament

Figure 23.3
The relations are shown between the retinacular ligament, the articular fibro-cartilage, and the accessory lateral ligament. The fibrous flexor tendon sheath is also shown.

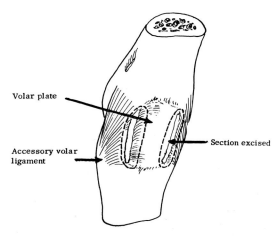

Volar plate

Accessory volar ligament

Section excised

Figure 23.5
The dotted lines indicate the area excised at the level of the volar plate and lateral accessory ligament.

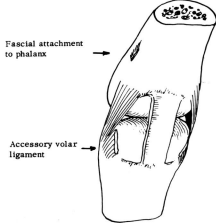

Fascial attachment to phalanx

Accessory volar ligament

Figure 23.6
Proximal interphalangeal joint, showing the proportions of the volar capsule and accessory ligaments to be excised. Note the phalangeal attachment of aponeurosis and the excised lateral ligament.

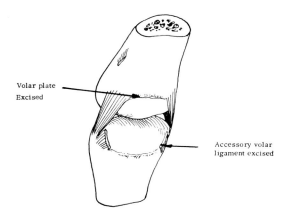

Figure 23.7
Diagram to show the total excision of the volar plate and accessory lateral ligaments.

Volar plate Excised

Accessory volar ligament excised

In several patients additional skin was needed. This was provided by a cross-finger pedicle flap in one case and a partial thickness skin graft in another.

SUMMARY

In a group of two hundred and twenty-two patients studied, the procedure of volar capsulectomy of the proximal interphalangeal joint was carried out in twenty-two patients. In those patients in whom volar capsulectomy of the proximal interphalangeal joint was carried out, an improvement in extension of this joint over that which had existed preoperatively was obtained in all instances. While complete extension of the finger was not obtained, it is felt by the author that this operative procedure is a worthwhile technique and may allow the operator to rehabilitate a finger which would otherwise be amputated. The operator must be cognizant of all the anatomical structures within the finger which may limit extension in a finger where flexion contracture is present in Dupuytren's contracture.

REFERENCES

CURTIS, R. M. (1954). Capsulectomy of the interphalangeal joints of the fingers, *Journal of Bone and Joint Surgery*, **36A**, 1219–1232.
HUESTON, J. T. (1963). *Dupuytren's Contracture*. Baltimore: Williams & Wilkins.

24. RECURRENCES IN DUPUYTREN'S CONTRACTURE

F. Iselin

By recurrence is meant the appearance of new aponeurotic lesions, either contracting or not, in an area where fasciectomy has been previously carried out for Dupuytren's contracture. This eliminates the recurrences of flexion deformity to 'false recurrences' which are due to operative complications rather than to a return of the disease process.

FALSE RECURRENCES

1. Scar contracture—this can be prevented by using modern techniques of exposure properly chosen and executed so that they will avoid sloughing of the skin.

2. Joint contracture—this is a consequence of the osteoarthritic dystrophy from postoperative swelling and retraction of the articular ligaments.

3. Extrinsic tendon imbalance—by failure to re-educate the extensor tendons postoperatively, these stretched and weakened tendons are readily overcome again by the powerful flexors which produce a return of flexion deformity in some cases. Thus a corrective splint to hold the finger in extension and assist the extensor tendon rehabilitation along with tranquillisers and exercises to overcome the dystrophy, and hormones if necessary to balance the protein components can all be brought to bear to reduce these causes of 'false recurrence'.

TRUE RECURRENCES

Hueston distinguished between recurrences and extensions in the postoperative course of Dupuytren's contracture—recurrences being the appearance of new lesions in an already operated area while extensions are the appearance of the lesions outside the operated area where previously no disease had been detectable. Thomine estimated the total frequency as about 29 per cent and pointed out that true recurrences were most frequent in the little finger and in the fingers were more important than in the palm while extensions in the thumb and the first web space were relatively innocuous.

A feature of these new lesions was their early appearance, being usually between 6 months and 2 years after the operation. Certain associated conditions such as Peronie's disease in young patients and being painful lesions all seemed to increase the incidence of recurrence of the condition.

We have treated, between 1962 and 1968, 33 cases of recurrence—of which only 9 were true recurrences. Four of these had been operated on initially by ourselves.

25. ENZYMIC FASCIOTOMY

John T. Hueston

It is 9 years since Bassot first reported his technique of 'exérèse pharmacodynamique' for Dupuytren's contracture—with illustrations of two patients whose gross flexion deformity had been completely corrected. In June 1969 he reported his results in 34 patients, again with illustrations of impressive corrections of severe deformities by this non-surgical method.

Therefore it appeared essential to investigate this alternative to surgery and to endeavour to place it in some perspective with relation to more orthodox surgical techniques.

In this method, trypsin is injected with local anaesthetic and hyaluronidase, at points along the length of the band and nodule. After 15 minutes, forcible extension is applied to rupture the deforming mechanism. We can confirm that in most cases virtually full passive extension can be obtained (Fig. 1).

Bassot's formula as published (1969) is—
Trypsine: 2·5 mg.
Alphachymotrypsine: 7·5 mg.
Hyaluronidase: 750 unites T.R.U.
Thiomucase: 300 unites T.R.A.
Ligocaine: 2 per cent; 20 ml.

The simplified formula we have been forced to use by unavailability of supplies has been—
Trypsin: 2·5 mg.
Hyaluronidase: B.P. 1500 units.
Xylocaine 2 per cent plain: 20 mls.

It is felt that much higher concentrations of trypsin can safely be used and in one of our cases 50 mg, was used over a multifocal palmar pattern of bands without any clinical evidence of neurological complications.

Multiple injections are made at each point chosen along the band and nodule. It may be suggested that this needling is in fact producing a traumatic or surgical fasciotomy; but controls with saline have failed to be effective.

On forcible extension, an audible cracking occurs, which is usually the palmar band being ruptured. The interphalangeal bands give the impression of stretching and tearing rather than frankly separating to leave such a palpable defect as is usual when the palmar band is ruptured. The correction is retained by a plaster slab for two to five days and then full movements are easily resumed. The plaster is used at night for two weeks.

Rupture of the skin has occurred in severely flexed cases with soft adherent skin in the flexure creases but although taking split-skin grafts readily, these defects have healed rapidly even when not grafted—as Bassot had already pointed out.

COMMENTARY

Bassot's reasoning is intensely logical—but it is probable that the process is simpler than he believes.

Planning his attack on what he regards as the essential

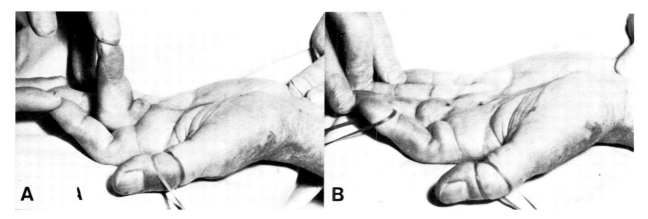

Figure 25.1
A, Dupuytren's contracture with 90° PIP flexion deformity of the middle finger and 40° PIP flexion deformity of the index. B, correction of the middle finger 15 minutes after enzymic injection.

three histological components of Dupuytren's contracture—fibroblastic proliferation, alteration and overproduction of ground substance and contraction of collagenous tissues—he mixes proteolytic and anti-inflammatory enzymes (trypsine and alphachymotrypsine) with enzymes to depolymerize and spread the ground substance (thiomucase and hyaluronidase) and lignocaine which, in addition to being local anaesthetic, may assist by decreasing the local reflex reaction ('neuroplegic' action).

Our investigations into the actual effect of this mixture on the tissues are based on (a) excision of the Dupuytren's tissue after injection and rupture, with histological studies, and (b) injection of recent cadaver material.

Macroscopically when the ruptured tissue is exposed the longitudinal fibres are seen to have been torn cleanly in the palm, leaving a lozenge shaped defect through which the intact synovial system of the flexor tendons can be seen (Fig. 25.2). There is little haemorrhage, partly because a tourniquet was almost immediately applied to allow resection of the specimen, and partly because only the poorly vascular band itself has been ruptured, with local oedema from the injection but little evidence of injury to adjacent tissues.

There is evidence of a regional injury over the following three to four days, with moderate swelling of the dorsum of the hand and of the injected finger—probably due partly to liberation of some tissue breakdown products from the enzyme action and partly purely traumatic. When exposure and formal fasciectomy has been proceeded with, the wound has had a more prolonged oedematous phase before final healing has occurred, as usual, at 2 weeks.

It is too soon to assess our personal series of 12 cases and since three of these have had immediate fasciectomies to provide tissue for study our material is very restricted.

While full metacarpophalangeal correction is the rule, there has been difficulty in obtaining sufficient traction on digital sections of the band, after the prior rupture of the palmar segment of the band to achieve rupture of the interphalangeal bands in three patients.

Bassot repeats his injections and traction on several occasions over a week or two until all residual bands have been eliminated. We have repeated the injections after one month for residual elements with some benefit.

Certainly full painless movements are present from two or three days after correction.

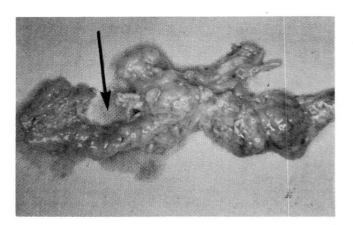

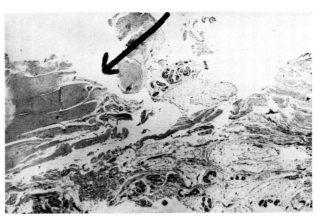

Figure 25.2
Operative specimen showing the rupture of the main longitudinal palmar band soon after enzymic fasciotomy. The rupture is surrounded by a moderate ecchymosis.

Figure 25.3
Longitudinal section at the point of aponeurotic rupture shown in Figure 25.2. Some debris has been introduced into the region of rupture during the preparation of the section.

Microscopically the margins of the point of rupture in the band appear to be staining normally with no cellular nuclear changes possibly because time has not been allowed for these to occur. Certainly there has been no instant massive chemical necrosis (Fig. 25.3).

Histological sections of cadaver muscle, tendon and nerve thus injected have shown no significant changes.

The trypsin is apparently at a safe concentration and the spreading agent insures that its action is likely to be measured in minutes rather than hours.

There has been no evidence of traction injury to digital nerves.

Rupture of the soft skin in the flexure creases after correction of severe deformity has been the major complication but its significance on the final result appears to be negligible.

From our findings it is suggested that 'enzymic fasciotomy' is a more accurate description of what occurs in this procedure than the 'pharmacodynamic excision' of Bassot.

There appears to be hardly any dissolution of tissue, but its main effect is to allow a facilitation of traumatic rupture. The consequences of rupture follow in much the same way as after a surgical rupture by fasciotomy.

COMMENT

Until much greater experience has been obtained with this method and an assessment of the late results has been made, the risk of advocating such a simple method is that many practitioners may attempt it without a full appreciation of the underlying condition of Dupuytren's contracture.

I would recommend its use in only a few selected instances, namely—

1. Where the patient is not medically fit even for regional anaesthesia, this local anaesthetic technique in the hand has allowed complete correction of metacarpophalangeal deformity.

2. Extensive multifocal disease in an elderly person where extensive surgery is preferably avoided.

3. In severe flexion deformity to provide metacarpophalangeal correction as a preliminary to a definitive fasciectomy of the fingers; that is to say in the same role

as Bunnell recommended preliminary surgical fasciotomy.

There is little reason to expect that this method will have any different effect than surgical fasciotomy on the disease process.

It is in the elderly with discrete mature bands that atrophy and apparently permanent resolution of the deforming mechanism is sometimes seen after accidental traumatic rupture or after a well performed fasciotomy. Shrinkage of digital nodules occurs when the longitudinal traction is relieved by fasciotomy and the recent recommendation by Gonzalez (that open digital transection of the deforming band-nodule mechanism be retained by insertion of a Wolfe graft), is based on his observation that resolution of the pathological process occurs on release of longitudinal tension.

It will require further study to determine whether these enzymes actually facilitate the natural resolution of the abnormal tissue in Dupuytren's contracture after release of the longitudinal tension.

CONCLUSION

Enzymic fasciotomy appears to offer an alternative to surgical fasciotomy in a few selected patients.

REFERENCES

BASSOT, J. (1965). Traitement de la maladie de Dupuytren par exérèse pharmacodynamique isolée ou complétée par un temps plastique uniquement cutane. *Lille Chirurgical* **XX,** No. 1.
BASSOT, J. (1969). Traitement de la maladie de Dupuytren par exérèse pharmacodynamique; bases physio-biologiques—technique. *Gazette des Hôpitaux* 557.

26. THE MANAGEMENT OF ECTOPIC LESIONS IN DUPUYTREN'S CONTRACTURE

John T. Hueston

One of the most fascinating aspects of Dupuytren's contracture is the occurrence, beyond the palm, of lesions histologically similar to those deposits classically recognized within the palm as Dupuytren's contracture. It is this frequent association of the palmar lesions with ectopic lesions that has led some surgeons to drop the more limited English term of Dupuytren's 'contracture' in preference for the more appropriate Dupuytren's 'disease' which is a broad enough term to include these other manifestations. It would appear that Dupuytren himself was aware that plantar lesions could occur, that a family can show inheritance of the condition and that it can occur in twins—but these general features of the disease are only included in the greatly expanded posthumously published second edition of his *Leçons Orales* in 1839 and were not in the original 1832 account.

With our increase in knowledge of the condition it is clear that only the minority of patients with Dupuytren's contracture do in fact manifest ectopic lesions and the most logical interpretation of the situation is to realize that the appearance and the extent of the ectopic deposits are helpful guides in the estimation of the severity of Dupuytren's 'diathesis' in any particular patient. It has been stressed in Chapter 11 of this monograph, that the timing and extent of surgery planned for any particular patient is largely based on an assessment of the strength of his predisposition to the production of this tissue—or diathesis—because this will help in the prediction of the likelihood of recurrences.

Of all the factors used in assessing the strength of a Dupuytren's diathesis the presence of ectopic deposits is probably the most important.

When considering aetiological questions in Dupuytren's contracture in Chapter 6 it was pointed out that the racial incidence of Dupuytren's contracture varies considerably and of course the incidence of ectopic deposits will likewise vary from one author to another if they are dealing with different populations. The incidence in the largely Celtic population of Melbourne was that of 159 patients requiring surgery for Dupuytren's contracture 19 showed plantar lesions, 67 showed knuckle pads and 5 showed penile lesions. Occasionally other rare sites have been observed such as along the subcutaneous tendons of flexor carpi ulnaris and flexor carpi radialis and the tendo Achilles.

NATURAL HISTORY OF ECTOPIC DEPOSITS

Ectopic lesions frequently confuse the unwary surgeon by appearing at an earlier age than the palmar lesions which are so well recognized as Dupuytren's contracture.

Thus, even if a surgeon is aware that Dupuytren's contracture in the palm may be associated with plantar nodules, the appearance of plantar masses in patients as young as 7 or 8 years—and often in girls—leads him often to operate on the foot rather than recognize that this is Dupuytren's contracture without as yet any hand lesions. Ultimately these young patients will develop typical palmar lesions and the general diathesis will be recognized. Tragedy has, however, sometimes befallen these youngsters because the clinical entity has not been recognized and a biopsy has likewise been incorrectly interpreted as fibrosarcoma and the leg has been amputated. The highly cellular nature of the fibroplastic histological pattern, frequently showing mitoses, is typical of ectopic lesions with only a gentle gradation to a lesser cellularity as we pass from foot to finger to penis and it is essential to interpret histological structure against the background of the patient as a whole, with particular regard to the Dupuytren's diathesis.

Knuckle pads over the dorsum of the proximal interphalangeal joints may appear first and have been seen along with plantar lesions in young patients still not showing any palmar lesions. More often one sees Dupuytren's contracture in only one palm but knuckle pads on one or more fingers of the opposite hand. These young patients with knuckle pads can be told confidently that sooner or later palmar lesions will appear and may require treatment. The youngest patient personally seen with knuckle pads was 14 years old and had a very strong family history of Dupuytren's contracture.

It is usual for the patients not to associate these dorsally situated digital lesions with the palmar lesions even when both are present and well developed. Many patients, as is notoriously common in their attempts to account for the commoner palmar lesion, will have some other explanation for the knuckle pads such as knocks on a car door or 'arthritis'. The only occupation which appears to produce a clinically similar dorsal callosity over the proximal interphalangeal joint is the slaughterman punching the skins off beasts in an abbatoir—and it is characteristic of the slaughterman's callosities that they diminish in size when he takes his annual vacation.

The penile lesion is in the wall of the corpora cavernosa and the later appearance of Dupuytren's contracture can be less confidently predicted in any particular individual because of the later age of onset of the penile lesions. It has been reported that of 85 patients with Peyronie's disease 8 had Dupuytren's contracture (Ciniewicz, 1956).

A feature of the ectopic lesions is that they may appear quite rapidly over the months but, once established, they often appear to remain stationary for many years. Curiously the histology does not show a great variety over the years and the same highly cellular active fibroplasia may comprise the bulk of a plantar lesion which has remained virtually unaltered in size for 20 years.

The other important clinical feature of the ectopic deposits is that they are not associated, except in the penis, with the progressive contracture and retraction that characterizes the palmar lesion. The penile lesions are sometimes associated with a circumferential constriction and certainly the disabling chordee on erection shows that some considerable infiltration and loss of local tissue elasticity has occurred.

It is probable that the relatively uniform histological fibroplastic picture may be related to the absence of contracture in these ectopic lesions if the 'extrinsic' theory of contraction in the palm is accepted rather than the 'intrinsic' theory—as was discussed in the chapter on aetiological questions. Thus the extensor mechanism in whose paratenon the lesion develops over the proximal interphalangeal joint is constantly stretched—as is also the denser plantar aponeurosis—so that there is less likelihood of these related anatomical structures being drawn up into the nodule to produce the combination histologically of juxtaposed mature fibrous tissue and active hypercellular areas.

MANAGEMENT OF ECTOPIC LESIONS

The absence of progressive contracture and a notoriously high and troublesome recurrence rate leads to the conclusion that surgery is not only unnecessary but contraindicated in most ectopic lesions.

Plantar lesions are usually quite painless and a mildly tender phase will usually pass in a few months. Only when a nodule has progressed to be several centimetres in diameter and constitutes a 'space-occupying lesion in the boot', need surgical reduction be considered. This feeling that there is a pebble in the shoe is uncommon but may be pressing enough to warrant relief. Such relief, however, may not be long-standing because recurrence and extension can both follow soon after the most careful dissection and resection of the nodule

and its related plantar aponeurosis (Fig. 26.1). A new field of peripheral nodules by extension can lead to worse symptoms than before the operative intervention and the prospect of repeated and increasingly extensive resection is unpleasant to confront. Fortunately the strong tendency to recurrence can—as in the palm—be controlled by free skin graft replacement of the related plantar skin.

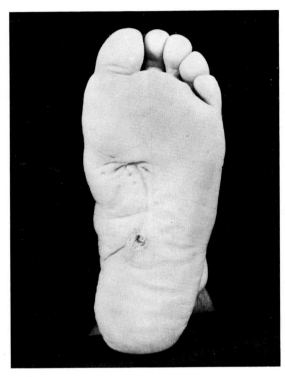

Figure 26.1
Local recurrence and significant extension of a plantar lesion with an ulcerated scarline following the excision of a 'sarcoma' at the age of 16 years. There has been little change in the past 24 years since this early recurrence. Five brothers are also severely affected with this disease and a twin has identical lesions in all four limbs to those of the patient illustrated.

Patients seen with increasingly widespread recurrences and the infliction of neuromata from surgical injury to plantar digital nerves—particularly when local excision has been repeated because of early reappearance of a mysterious mass, often still undiagnosed—has led to an extremely conservative approach to these plantar ectopic lesions.

The knuckle pads also may be tender during their appearance but later only cause discomfort if accidentally knocked. It is unusual for a patient to request their removal unless they have appeared before the palmar Dupuytren's contracture and there has been raised some fear of arthritis or malignancy. They are much less common in women than are plantar lesions and hence their removal on aesthetic grounds is rarely requested. Sometimes, however, disfigurement and nuisance value combine to warrant excision of these lesions.

A very high recurrence rate is found after excision of these knuckle pads and, as also after excision of plantar lesions, the recurrences appear within a few months and may be more tender and troublesome than the original lesion. Fortunately it has been found in this situation also that recurrence can be prevented by free skin graft replacement of the area overlying the proximal inter-phalangeal joint region—corresponding to the elipse enclosed between the most distal and the most proximal transverse dorsal skin wrinkles in this area.

Non-operative management is likewise advised when knuckle pads are found at unusual sites such as over the interphalangeal joint of the thumb of the distal inter-phalangeal joint region—corresponding to the ellipse digits.

In general, explanation and reassurance are enough to allow the patient to accept and live with knuckle pads and with plantar lesions.

Impotence is the usual presenting symptom with advanced Peyronie's disease but impotence is also the usual aftermath of surgical resection of Peyronie's disease. In the preoperative state the impotence is due to a deforming degree of chordee, sometimes painful, but psychologically this difficulty is far less damaging to the patient's male ego than the flaccid impotence which is seen after resection. Injections of hydrocortis-one into the plaque usually require a general anaesthetic if they are to be adequate in volume and precise in place-ment. This frequently allows some improvement although rarely a cure, but it appears that such a non-surgical procedure—by not interfering with the integrity of the tunica of the corpora, retains the normal physiological pressure systems essential for erection.

SUMMARY

Plantar lesions and knuckle pads are to be sought in all patients with Dupuytren's contracture as providing useful information for the assessment of the Dupuy-tren's diathesis on which treatment can then be planned.

They may often precede the palmar lesions of Dupuy-tren's contracture and lead to diagnostic confusion and even tragedy. Freedom from contraction and deformity makes surgery rarely needed except if a lesion is extremely large.

A very high recurrence rate makes surgery usually futile and often increases the disability rather than relieves it.

Free skin graft replacement is found to prevent recurrence in ectopic sites as it has previously been shown in the palm.

REFERENCES

Ciniewicz, O. W. (1961). *Lancet*, i, 622.
Hueston, J. T. (1963). *Dupuytren's Contracture*. Edinburgh: Living-stone.

27. THE TREATMENT OF PEYRONIE'S DISEASE BY METHYLHYDRAZINE

E. Benassayag

As a coincidental observation during the treatment of a patient with Hodgkin' disease using methylhydrazine, it was also noted that the Dupuytren's contracture in the palm of the same patient was relieved or at least improved. This observation which was reported by Aron in 1968 aroused our interest in the related condition of Peyronie's disease where we have attempted to follow on his interesting observation.

We would like to report here the result of this clinical trial.

Many studies have been made on Peyronie's disease, clinical radiological and therapeutic. We will not dwell on the clinical aspects but merely point out its characteristics which are—the variable distribution, with, however, a common result namely a painful deviation of the penis:

the variable age incidence;

the failed radiological attempts to demonstrate the fibrous lesions;

the multiplicity of forms of treatment which have been proposed.

VARIABILITY OF THE LESIONS

The situation and the extent of the fibrous process involving the corpora cavernosa is usually self-evident.

There may be a single lesion or multiple lesions, an irregular involvement, bilateral or unilateral and it may be symmetrical or not and occur from the root of the penis up to the glans. An irregular patchy distribution may occur or a continuous total fibrosis involving the whole extent of both corpora cavernosa.

On erection two deformities appear—an angulation of the penis at the level of the indurated plaque drawing down the shaft of the organ into an angle even beyond a right angle, the deviation being sometimes dorsal or sometimes lateral—and a constriction of the shaft of the penis at the level of the induration so that a dumbell appearance is produced.

These deformities are generally extremely painful.

Intercourse is difficult, added to which is a partial or total impotence despite some persisting early morning erections which although useless are still painful.

THE NATURAL HISTORY

This must be known before being able to judge the efficiency of any treatment. J. L. Williams and C. J. Thomas have in 1968 reported 21 cases of which 12

had no treatment and 9 were submitted to between 600 and 1500 rad of X-ray therapy in 6 doses. Over a period of several months or years it was possible to observe a spontaneous improvement. The improvement was in the order first of the disappearance of the pain and then the plaque and then the penile deviation. No difference was noted between those patients which had been irradiated and those which had not been irradiated. Out of the 21 cases 6 had been totally cured and 10 improved, sufficient to allow the resumption of sexual intercourse, and 5 showed no improvement at all. The average time for complete healing was about 4 years. The duration therefore of any treatment must be always reported along with the treatment if one is going to claim to have been able to improve on the healing of the condition.

METHYLHYDRAZINE

At first we should be familiar with the possibilities, the repercussions or the dangers of such a product. The anti-tumoural properties of methylhydrazine have been well established as a result of its being a very active cytostatic agent. We have used the chlorhydrate derivative p-(N-methylhydrazinomethyl)-N-isopropyl benzamide.*

TOXICITY

The absolute toxicity has been studied by the lethal dose for 50 per cent of experimental animals and has been established at between 700 and 1400 milligrams per kilogram weight.

The sublethal toxicity studied over several weeks has shown that a dose of 20 milligrams per kilogram allows animals to remain alive and in good health.

The lethal dose in one week was 200 milligrams per kilogram. It produced at first a white cell depression and lack of resistance to infection. The leucocytes and particularly the polymorphs were most affected and then the lymphocytes. The platelets were slightly less susceptible and the erythrocytes were hardly affected at all.

Histological examination of the tissues of animals dying from this product have shown a moderate amount of liver damage, and testicular damage particularly in

* Natulan (Roche).

germinal epithelium but scarcely any other tissue damage was noted.

MODE OF ACTION

This is complex because there is a reduction of the mitotic index and prolongation of the interphase in cellular division with changes and fragmentation of chromatin.

Biochemically the changes were similar to those from ionizing irradiation (alcoylants).

In addition some notable changes also follow the action of this drug.

1. An inhibition of monoaminoxydase. This is in common with all the I.M.A.O. but is must less than that produced by iproniazide from which it has been derived. There is a potentiation of other drugs with this central action namely reinforcement and prolongation of the effects of chlorpromazine and the barbiturates.

2. A moderate elevation of the blood sugar so that it is necessary to take special precautions when treating diabetics.

3. Its action on the metabolism of alcohol produces a dysulfirane type of 'flush syndrome'.

4. There is a slight increase in the pulse and respiration rates and occasionally a slight elevation of blood pressure.

Generally the tolerance is good but one should be prepared for the possibility of certain side-effects.

1. Bowel disturbances. These do not last through the whole course of treatment, usually commencing with the treatment but disappearing in the second week and mainly presenting as nausea, anorexia and more rarely as flatulence or vomiting. These troubles can be minimized or even eliminated by taking the drug either during or immediately after a meal and using vitamin B_6, antiemetics, antihistamines or antacids.

2. Skin disturbances are rare but may be allergic rashes urticaria or eczematous and in these cases it will be better to stop the treatment.

3. Blood disturbances are less severe than one would at first suspect. In fact like all the cytostatic drugs, methylhydrazine does inhibit haematopoeisis but much less than radiotherapy or other agents which are usually used in higher doses in the region of 6 to 8 grams.

The blood changes are essentially a leukopenia, affecting mainly the polymorphs, but reversible in one or two weeks after cessation of treatment, which can then be started again without risk of more rapid deterioration of the blood picture. A tendency to eosinophilia has been noted but the erythrocytes are rarely disturbed except for occasional anisocytosis with poikilocytosis.

4. Other secondary effects have occasionally been seen, such as congestion of the face and ears simulating a 'flush' syndrome following alcohol. Giddiness, general aching and loss of weight have been noted after taking alcohol or cytotropic drugs during treatment but if these are avoided the methylhydrazine appears to be quite safe.

Dosage starting with 150 milligrams capsule per day for 2 or 3 weeks and then 2 capsules per day, the treatment can after 2 or 3 months be stopped for two weeks and then commenced again at 2 capsules each of 100 milligrams per day.

The duration of the treatment depends on the results.

Higher doses can also be used up to even 6 or 7 capsules per day but such treatment should be stopped after a total of 7 or 8 weeks.

A drop in the white cell count to 3000 or in the platelets to 100,000 is an indication to stop treatment and it is then necessary to carry out a regular review of the blood picture every two weeks. It is clear that such treatment as this should not be used in people with pre-existing bone marrow disease but this has not been found to be associated at all commonly with Peyronie's disease.

One excludes for the same reason those patients with renal or liver disease or unstable diabetes.

TOLERANCE AND EFFICIENCY

We have studied 17 cases ranging in age from 25 to 71 years. The duration of the disease before beginning treatment was from 2 months to 20 years. The general tolerance of the drug has been good in all cases. Some digestive troubles were noted—one case of diarrhoea which cleared up 3 days after stopping treatment, three cases of nausea and one case of constipation.

The haematological tolerance has been good in 14 cases—but two cases developed a leukopenia of 3800 and 3500 both of which returned to normal within 10 days of stopping treatment, one case of relative (35 per cent granulocytopenia without leukopenia also cleared up ten days after cessation of treatment.

In these 3 cases there was no infection during the phase of blood disturbance and treatment was recommenced without further trouble.

EFFICACY

The first sign of improvement appeared within 3 to 5 weeks then became quite obvious.

First there was a loss of pain on erection, then a diminution in the deviation of the penis and one angulation which had previously exceeded 90 degrees became almost straight, the penis straightening itself progressively although not becoming absolutely straight. The most important improvement was that sexual intercourse became once more possible.

At the same time but rather more slowly the transverse constriction at the level of the plaque in the corpora cavernosa became less.

Along with this improvement the fibrous plaque itself was noted to become softer during the first month and later stretch and become more supple and at times even to fragment—but particularly it diminished in volume both in extent and in thickness.

At the beginning of the treatment the corpora cavernosa appeared at first to be harder and thicker as though the penis was shrunken on itself like a telescope and it was necessary to manipulate it a little to really appreciate the changes.

RESULTS

We can report 10 cures, three significant improvements, three moderate improvements and one failure.

The cures occurred: two in $2\frac{1}{2}$ months, one in 3 months, four in 4 months and one at 8 months.

By a cure we mean total disappearance of the induration, the deviation and the deformity.

Three cases of significant improvement, almost complete disappearance of the deformity and of the plaque was noted and the treatment is continuing.

In three cases despite treatment for 4 months in two cases and 7 months in the third, evident improvement has been obtained but not sufficient for sexual satisfaction.

Finally one total failure occurred with actual increase in the volume of the fibrous plaque.

We present this work as the basis of some studies in the treatment of an ill-understood disease admittedly benign but much more incapacitating than is usually realized.

REFERENCES

ARON, E. (1968). Le traitement medical de la maladie de Dupuytren par un agent cytostatique. *Presse médicale,* **76,** 1956.

WILLIAMS, J. L. & THOMAS, C. G. (1968). Natural history of la Peyronie's disease. Proceedings of the Royal Society of Medicine, **61,** 876–877.

BOULKER, P. & BENASSAYAG, E. (1970). Traitement de la maladie de la Peyronie par la methylhydrazine. In: *64ᵉ Congres français d'Urologie, Paris,* 1970.

28. THE PALMAR FASCIA, AND THE DEVELOPMENT OF DEFORMITIES AND DISPLACEMENTS IN DUPUYTREN'S CONTRACTURE*

H. Graham Stack

The Hunterian lectures were instituted to do honour to John Hunter, who by his work, his writings, and his collection of specimens laid the scientific foundations of modern surgery. He left no specimen of contracture of the fingers, and I can find no reference to the condition in his writings.

The earliest mention I have been able to find is made by Felix Plater of Basel, who died in 1614. In his *Observations* published in 1641, he reported the case of a quarry worker, considered that it was due to retraction of the tendons, and attributed the condition to turning immense stones (Plater, 1641). The first written report that the condition was due to contracture of the palmar fascia was that made by Astley Cooper in 1822 (Cooper, 1822). Astley Cooper was a pupil of Hunter's, and is described as having been able to take Hunter's principles and project them into successful practical surgery (Brock, 1952). However, there is no doubt that the first full description of the condition and its treatment is that of Baron Dupuytren, in his *Leçons Orales*, published in 1832, and it is as Dupuytren's contracture that the condition is known throughout the world (Dupuytren, 1832).

The first important review of the anatomy of this area was written by Maslieurat-Lagémard in 1839 (Maslieurat-Lagémard, 1839). He was assistant to Cruveilhier, the Professor of Anatomy at the Hôtel Dieu, where Dupuytren was the chief surgeon. His paper makes mention of the discussions, obviously sometimes quite controversial, which had taken place there. Maslieurat-Lagémard appreciated that the palmar aponeurosis made a continuous sheet as it thinned out to cover the flexor tendon sheaths, and he also described the arcade of fibres running down into the fingers which we now call the superficial transverse ligaments of the palm.

Cleland of Glasgow described the cutaneous ligament of the finger as a strong band arising mainly from the lateral ridges of the proximal phalanx and running to the skin, the main function being to maintain the position of the skin of the fingers (Cleland, 1878).

Grapow (1887) recognized the formation of sheets of fascia, particularly the continuity of the flexor retinaculum and the transverse fibres. He noted the multiple attachments of the longitudinal layer distally to the natatory ligaments, to the periosteum and to the bone,

and through the fat to the skin, particularly in the neighbourhood of the flexion creases.

Legueu and Juvara (1892) also recognized that the fascias existed in sheets, and distinguished the three transverse layers: the transverse fibres of the palmar aponeurosis, the superficial transverse ligaments of the palm, and the deep aponeurotic layer, the anterior interosseous fascia.

From these writings it emerged that the fascia can be regarded as occurring in sheets, each layer of fascia covering a layer of muscle or tendons. In this context, the longitudinal layer, the continuation of the palmaris longus muscle, is regarded as a tendinous layer (Landsmeer, 1956).

Clinical observation of cases of Dupuytren's contracture has always revealed great variability in the physical signs and it has been suggested, most recently by Hueston in his Hunterian Lecture in 1963 (Hueston, 1965), that the distribution of the contractures does not follow an anatomical pattern.

Harvey Allen (1954) used to demonstrate what he called the spiralling of the nerves around the contracted bands, describing the work of his colleague Michael Mason. Iselin (1955), Hueston (1963), and Gosset (1966) have all illustrated the mechanism. Difficulty has arisen during operations due to the displacements of the digital nerves, which may be very difficult to find. It is the intention of this study to show that the anatomical distribution of the fibres varies in such a way that it is possible to explain all the different clinical forms of the disease, and to predict when the digital nerves will be displaced.

MATERIAL

SERIAL SECTIONS

Examination was made of serial sections of foetal hands from embryos of about 16 to 18 weeks of foetal life. Several series were examined both transverse, longitudinal and frontal. In the present investigations the

* This article which is the text of the Hunterian Lecture was first printed in the *Annals of the Royal College of Surgeons of England*, vol. 48, pp. 238–251 (April 1971). It is reproduced here with the kind permission of the Editor.

A monograph on this subject is published by Churchill Livingstone entitled *The Palmar Fascia*.

following series of sections in the Anatomical Department of the University of Leiden have been examined:

	Series number	Embryo size (cm)	Age
Two transverse	1452	22	22 weeks
Two frontal	1900	14	
	1931	11	16 to 18 weeks
	1928	13	
One sagittal	1901	14	

Several series of sections prepared by Dr K. M. Backhouse were also examined.

The sections are 10 μm in thickness (10 μm per section = 100 sections per mm) and are mounted on numbered slides. There are approximately 4000 sections to each transversely cut hand. The illustrations are made from slides stained with Azan.

DISSECTION

It must be remembered that dissection consists essentially of the removal of connective tissue, and that the dissection of fascia is largely the destruction of the tissue under examination. However, many dissections have been carried out over a considerable period of time, some in cadavers, and many during surgical operations. The author has experience of over 300 dissections of the palmar fascia in cases of Dupuytren's contracture.

Fig. 28.1 shows a cross section of the palm of the right hand, between the middle and the ring metacarpals. The middle metacarpal head is on the left and the ring on the right. The cut has been made somewhat obliquely so that it passes through the ring metacarpal rather more distally. A small piece of the base of the proximal phalanx is visible close to the ring metacarpal. The top of the picture is dorsal. At the bottom is the palmar skin, with the distal palmar crease indenting it.

On the lateral side of the metacarpal heads lie the collateral ligaments of the metacarpophalangeal joints, and these merge anteriorly with the volar plates. In the

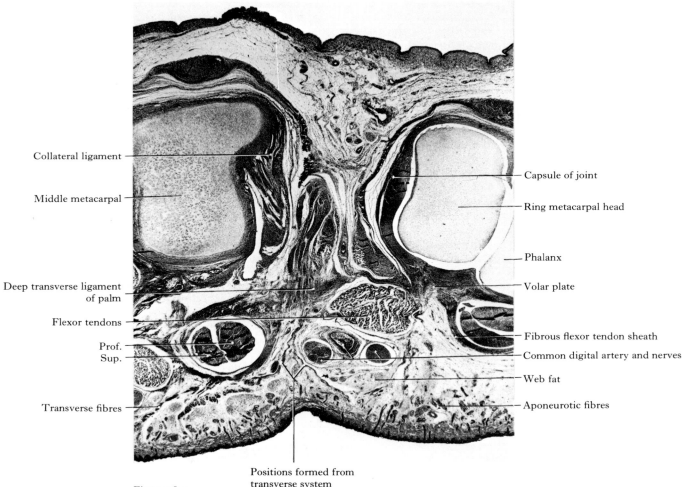

Figure 28.1

A cross section of the palm of the right hand, between the middle and the ring metacarpals.

ring finger the volar plate is a dense wedge of tissue, which is attached to the base of the proximal phalanx, and the flexor tendons lie on it, secured by the fibrous flexor tendon sheath. In the middle finger the volar plate is represented by two folds of tissue, part attached to the neck of the bone, and the free part of the plate lying close to the tendons.

Stretching horizontally across the figure between the two volar plates is the deep transverse ligament of the palm. This merges proximally with the anterior interosseous fascia, and separates the interosseous muscles from the flexor tendons and the lumbrical muscles.

Here the lumbrical muscle can be seen lying between the volar plate and the common palmar digital artery and the digital nerves. Between the vessels and the skin lies a small oval of fat, the commencement of the fat pad of the web.

Behind the volar plate can be seen the terminations of the interosseous muscles and their tendons, joining the extensor expansions which lie on the dorsum of the metacarpal heads.

If the reader pays particular attention to the flexor tendon sheath in front of the middle metacarpal on the left side of the picture, it will be seen that there is a row of oval bundles of fibres, stretching from the edge of the figure to merge intimately with the tendon sheath itself. They represent the obliquely cut fibres of the transverse fibres of the palmar aponeurosis, sometimes called the superficial palmar ligament (Skoog, 1967).

These fibres merge proximally with the flexor retinaculum and distally are contiguous with, or possibly even continuous with, the fibrous flexor tendon sheath.

More superficially to these fibres, lying between the fibrous flexor tendon sheath and the subcutaneous fat and the skin, there is another layer of transversely cut fibres. These represent the pretendinous languette of the middle finger, the longitudinal continuation of the palmar aponeurosis proper.

They form a ribbon-like band lying in front of the flexor tendons. On the medial side of the tendon sheath a clearly marked fibre passes from this band backwards and medially between the flexor tendon sheath and the digital nerve. This is the standard pattern that can be seen throughout the series. This fibre passes to be inserted into the deep transverse ligament of the palm.

Fig. 28.2: The basic pattern of this figure is the same. On the left is the middle finger metacarpal. In the ring

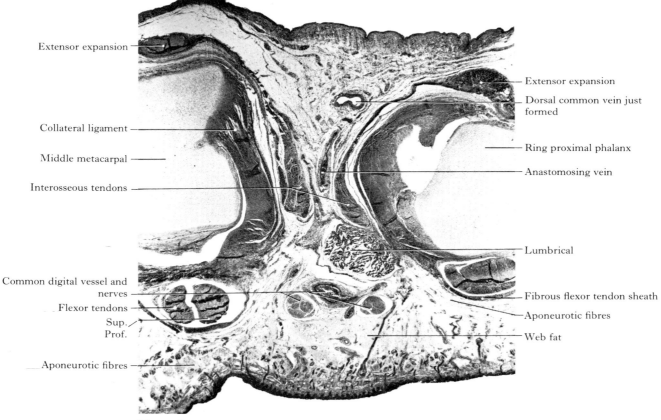

Figure 28.2
The basic pattern of this figure is the same as that of Figure 28.1.

finger the bone seen is the base of the proximal phalanx. The flexor tendons lie directly on the surface of the bone. In the middle finger the tendons are separated from the bone by the volar plate.

We are now beyond the point where the deep transverse ligament of the palm is in continuity, but at the same point on the figure there is a dense mass of tissue which lies close to the lumbrical giving rise to a ring of fibrous tissue embracing the muscle and holding it to the base of the phalanx. This mass of tissue corresponds to the site of the proximal extension of Cleland's ligament.

On the extreme left of the figure anterior to the fibrous flexor tendon sheath can be seen the two layers of bundles of fascia. The transverse fibres lie nearer to the sheath, and more superficially are the fibres of the languette, obvious only on the radial side. On the ulnar side the strong fibres are not so obvious, but there is a streaming effect of fibres passing between the fibrous flexor tendon sheath and the digital nerve, towards the side of the volar plate, and towards the central bundle of fibres mentioned before.

Lying just beneath the skin on the volar surface some horizontally running fibres can be seen contributing to the increased thickness of the skin. This is the commencement of the superficial transverse ligament of the palm.

Fig. 28.3: The level of this figure is more distal than the metacarpal heads, and a deep cleft is showing in the dorsal skin. The bone in each finger is the proximal phalanx: in the middle finger the cartilaginous base of the bone is seen, and in the ring finger there is the cortical bone of the shaft. In both fingers the flexor tendons are lying directly on the bone.

The common digital artery has divided into two, and each digital nerve has just given off its dorsal branch.

The languettes of the palmar aponeurosis have thinned out by this level, and this layer is represented by the streaming fibres between the fibrous flexor tendon sheath and the nerves and vessels on each side.

Dorsally this stream of fibres is passing towards the skin fold and this is particularly noticeable on the middle finger.

The superficial fascia, the superficial transverse

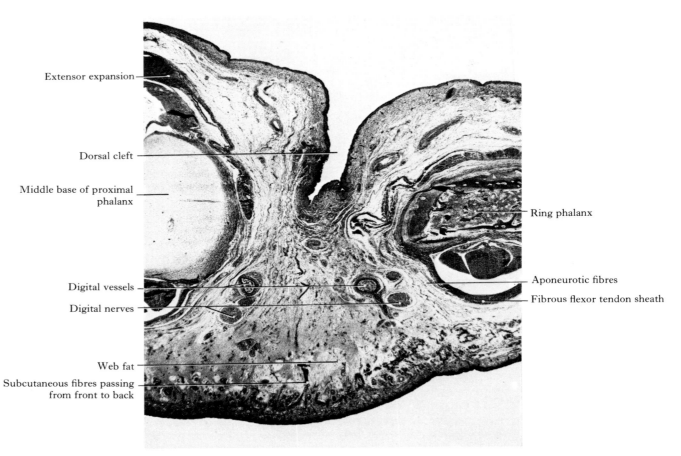

Figure 28.3
A cross section at the level of the bases of the proximal phalanges.

ligaments of the palm are seen here as a mass of tissue lying directly beneath the skin, particularly in front of the tendons and vessels.

Right in the centre of the figure, where the fat pad is causing prominence of the skin, there is a very thick dark fibre which passes backwards. There are several fibres of this nature passing dorsally between the neuro-vascular bundles. This is the general direction of many fibres of the superficial layer, forming the distal boundary of the web space. Their ultimate destination will be like the longitudinal layer, the mid-lateral line of the finger.

Fig. 28.4: In this figure the two fingers are almost

Fibres of this system are also seen passing in the remaining fragment of the web to join similar fibres in the other finger. These are the most distal fibres of the superficial transverse ligaments of the palm forming the support of the web, sometimes called the natatory ligament.

Thus we have now seen the general direction of the two main layers of the fascia, the longitudinal layer passing dorsally between the flexor tendon sheath and the vessels, and the superficial layer passing dorsally on the other side of the vessels, the two layers making a sling between which the neurovascular bundle lies. Both these layers pass to the mid-lateral line of the

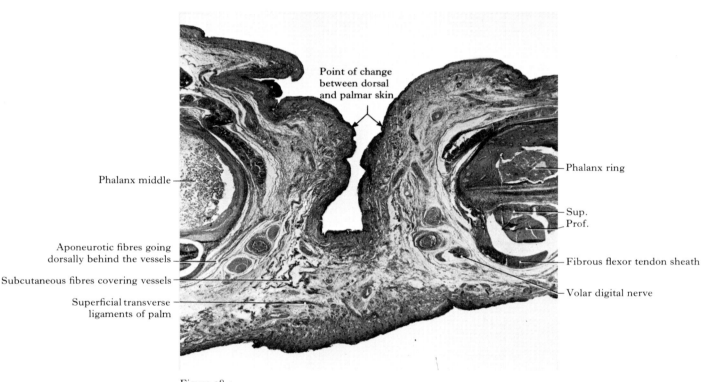

Figure 28.4
The two fingers are almost separated, only a small piece of the web

separated, only a small piece of the web remaining. The fibres of the longitudinal layer are still visible as parallel streams of fibres covering the fibrous flexor tendon sheath, and passing between the sheaths and the digital nerves and vessels. Dorsally the fibres pass towards the skin, particularly to the mid-lateral line of the fingers.

The superficial fibres are markedly in evidence in the middle finger running from the subcutaneous area in front of the tendon sheath, covering the vessels and passing to the mid-lateral line of the finger, here just dorsal to the skin cleft.

finger, and intermingle with Cleland's ligaments.

Fig. 28.5: This shows a longitudinal section through the centre of a middle finger. The bones are, from left to right, the metacarpal, and the proximal phalanx. Anterior to the middle metacarpal is a mass of interosseous muscle. Lying on the distal part of this muscle is a fragment of lumbrical, and over the proximal part is the base of the thenar muscle mass.

In front of the metacarpal head lie the volar plate and the long flexor tendons. The median nerve shows at two points: in the centre of the thenar mass, where the thenar branch is arising, and immediately anterior to

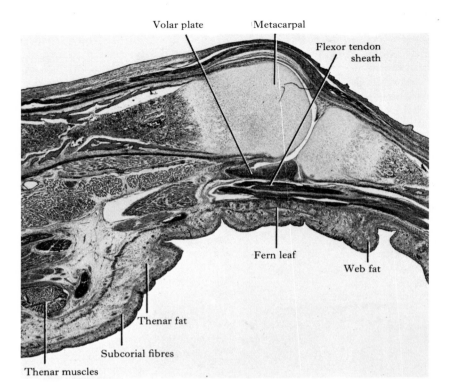

Volar plate | Metacarpal | Flexor tendon sheath

Fern leaf

Web fat

Thenar fat

Subcorial fibres

Thenar muscles

the fragment of lumbrical muscle.

In the triangle of pale tissue between these two fragments of nerve and the skin there is a dark line. This is the palmar part of the longitudinal layer of the palmar aponeurosis. As it passes distally it comes to lie close over the median nerve, and the deep cleft above it here is the thenar crease. Beyond this crease, in front of the metacarpal head, are the proximal and distal palmar creases, and in front of the proximal half of the proximal phalanx there is a deep bifid cleft which represents the palmo-digital crease.

If the reader will now pay particular attention to the area between proximal and distal palmar creases, and the flexor tendon sheath and the skin, the longitudinal fibres of the palmar aponeurosis will be seen as a dense line, and there are two rows of condensed tissue in front of and behind this line. This material together forms a pattern like a fern leaf. The condensed bundles represent the fibres passing forwards and backwards from the longitudinal layer.

Forwards they pass to be attached to the deep surface of the skin, and backwards they pass on either side to be attached to the sides of the fibrous flexor tendon sheaths, and to the sides of the phalanx. These fibres form the main deep attachment of the longitudinal layer.

Fig. 28.6 shows these structures diagramatically.

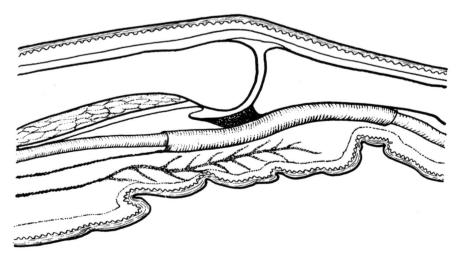

Figure 28.6
A diagrammatic illustration of the structures in Figure 28.5.

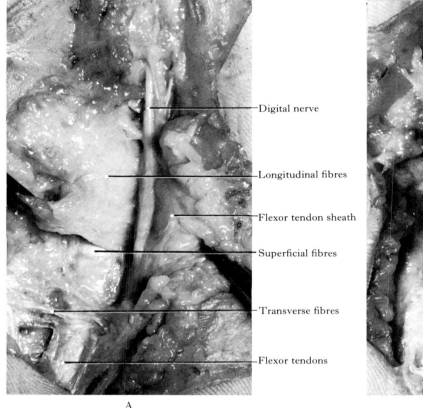

Digital nerve

Longitudinal fibres

Flexor tendon sheath

Superficial fibres

Transverse fibres

Flexor tendons

Skin attachment of Cleland's ligament

Digital band

Flexor tendons

Pin in M.P. joint space

Digital nerve

Anterior interosseous fascia

Lumbrical muscle

A

B

Figure 28.7
A, B, dissection of the ring finger of a left hand.

Fig. 28.7: Two illustrations of a dissection of the ring finger of a left hand are shown. The top of the figures is distal.

Fig. 28.7A: The skin has been turned down through a sinuous longitudinal incision. The superficial transverse ligament of the palm has been divided and turned over to the right. The pretendinous languette of the longitudinal fibres has been divided and turned distally and to the left, exposing the transverse fibres of the palmar aponeurosis proximally. Between these fibres and the turned-down longitudinal fibres, a small triangular piece of the fibrous flexor tendon sheath is visible and the form of the tendons can be seen lying beneath. The ulnar digital nerve to the ring finger runs up the centre of the figure, and the fact that the longitudinal fibres of the palmar aponeurosis pass as a sheet dorsally and more obliquely between the fibrous flexor tendon sheaths and the digital nerve can be seen.

The superficial layer also passes dorsally, between the digital nerves to the two fingers, the radial digital nerve to the little finger lying unexposed to the right of the picture.

Fig. 28.7B: The second illustration shows a deeper stage of the dissection. The superficial layer, the longitudinal layer, and the transverse fibres have all been removed.

The digital nerve has been retracted to the left, and the flexor tendon sheath divided, exposing the flexor tendons. One pin retracts the lumbrical muscle of the little finger to the right. The other pin is inserted in the metacarpophalangeal joint to show its level, and to hold the tendons back. This exposes the anterior interosseous fascia and the volar plate, and arising from this layer is a strong band of fibres, running distally and ulnarwards. At the top right-hand corner of the picture these fibres join the skin and the remainder of Cleland's ligament.

DISPOSITION OF THE LAYERS

These findings confirm that the fascial layers can be regarded as continuous sheets, covering each layer of muscles or tendons.

The anterior interosseous fascia covers the interosseous muscles, and distally is continuous with the volar plates and the deep transverse ligaments of the palm, and more distally still in the fingers with Cleland's ligaments, or the digital band (Thomine, 1965).

The flexor tendons and the lumbricals lie on this layer, and are covered by the flexor retinaculum, the transverse fibres of the palmar aponeurosis and the fibrous flexor tendon sheaths.

The next tendinous layer has been modified to become the palmar aponeurosis, arising from the palmaris longus.

Over this is the superficial layer which in the palm is mainly the subcorial fibrous tissue, thickened in the distal palm as the superficial transverse ligament of the palm, and more distally as the superficial fascia of the fingers.

ATTACHMENTS

The attachments of the various layers can be summarized as follows:

Deep layer to the periosteum of the metacarpals, to the volar plates and the deep transverse ligaments of the palm. The distal part becomes the digital band and is attached to the mid-lateral line of the fingers.

Transverse layer. Arising proximally as the flexor retinaculum, it is fused with the other fascias over the thenar and hypothenar muscles. Distally it fuses with the fibrous flexor tendon sheaths.

Longitudinal layer. Arising from the palmaris longus tendon, it divides into pretendinous languettes. Each of these sends fibres forwards to attach to the deep surface of the palmar skin, particularly in the region of the palmar creases. Posteriorly it sends an arcade of fibres backwards on each side of the flexor tendon sheaths. The majority of these fibres only arise beyond the level of the palmar creases, at the distal edge of the transverse fibres of the palmar aponeurosis, though a few may pass posteriorly by piercing these fibres.

The arcade fibres are attached to each side of the metacarpophalangeal joints, to the sides of the proximal phalanges, and to some extent to the middle phalanges. Rarely a few of these fibres may reach the distal phalanx.

Some of the fibres of the longitudinal layer pass backwards between the fibrous flexor tendon sheaths and the vessels to approach the mid-lateral line of the digit to fuse with the digital band.

The superficial layer. The proximal palmar part of this layer is closely attached to the back or deep surface of the skin, as the subcorial fibres. In the metacarpophalangeal part of the palm this layer is represented by the superficial transverse ligaments of the palm, which stretch across the palm from side to side. These fibres are closely attached to the skin throughout, particularly to the palmo-digital creases, and also to the anteromedial and antero-lateral borders of the fingers running distally from the webs.

The superficial fascial layer of the fingers covers the fingers from side to side between these borders, and then passes backwards to join the other fascial layers and the digital bands at the mid-lateral line of the fingers.

RESULTS OF CONTRACTURE OF THE LAYERS

The transverse fibres and the fibrous flexor tendons sheaths are never involved in contracture, unless it is occasionally by direct involvement due to extensive disease of one of the other layers (Skoog, 1967).

The longitudinal layer undergoes contracture by very firm fibrous strands. The forward-going fibres reach the skin and by contracture cause skin tether and sometimes deep pits. Contracture of the main longitudinal strands give rise to the strong bands which raise the skin and flex the fingers. These strands may be attached to any of the phalanges, usually the proximal phalanx, often the middle phalanx, and very occasionally the distal phalanx. These are the usual bands which cause contracture of the fingers.

Contracture of the longitudinal fibres which pass between the fibrous flexor tendon sheaths and the digital nerves and vessels, and become attached to the skin of the mid-lateral line, cause flexion of the fingers, like the previous category, but also cause deep skin tether and cause displacement of the digital nerve which is found crossing the strands from the web space towards the axis of the finger.

The posterior arcade fibres sometimes give rise to very strong thick bands passing backwards to the anterior interosseous fascia and the metacarpals. These are usually distal to the transverse fibres, but occasionally pierce them. They cause deep tethering of the whole aponeurosis.

The superficial fibres. Affection of these fibres by the disease is often of the fibrous nodular form distinguished by Nezelof and Tubiana (1958). In these cases the tissue is closely applied to the skin. Where these fibres of the superficial transverse ligaments of the palm pass into the fingers at the anteromedial and anterolateral borders of the fingers, there is often considerable tension under the skin, between the web, and the skin on the side of the proximal interphalangeal joints. This form of the disease also causes interdigital contracture preventing two fingers from being separated.

Digital band contracture. Occasionally the digital band running from the volar plates towards the mid-lateral line of the fingers may be involved. There is then a thickened band closely applied to the skin of the finger as far as or beyond the proximal interphalangeal joint. This can often cause intractable contracture of the finger, and is often responsible for the inability to extend the proximal interphalangeal joint, even after removal of the more common central strands of the longitudinal layer. This strand must be carefully sought for in all cases. It is often exposed and divided in the preparation of the lateral incisions when performing a z-plasty.

There is also a rare form of displacement of the digital nerve by the involvement of this layer pushing a digital nerve forward into a position of danger.

DIGITAL NERVE DISPLACEMENT

Fig. 28.8A illustrates a case of Dupuytren's contracture affecting the little finger. There was a contracture of the finger affecting mainly the metacarpophalangeal joint, though the proximal interphalangeal joint was also flexed to some extent.

The main strand was palpable raising the skin, and passing towards the radial side of the finger. It was predicted that the digital nerve would probably be found involved by the strand. Fig. 28.8B shows the same case at operation. The strand was exposed through an L-shaped incision, the transverse limb in the distal palmar crease, and the vertical limb in the midline of the finger.

Two strands were found, a strong one on the radial side with the radial digital nerve crossing it and also a weaker central strand passing to the middle phalanx, and not involving the nerve.

PREDICTION OF NERVE DISPLACEMENT

In a case where a longitudinal strand arising from the palmar triangle approaches a finger towards one or other side, and gains attachment to the skin in the mid-lateral line, it may be expected that the digital nerve will be caught up, and cross the strand from the web space towards the middle of the finger.

RESULTS

During the 10-year period 1959–1969, 237 operations were carried out on 204 patients, and during this time 29 displacements were seen.

SUMMARY

The attachments and the distribution of the layers of the palmar fascia have been studied in foetal serial sections and by dissection. Clinical evaluation of many cases of Dupuytren's contracture has been made. The findings have clearly confirmed that the fascia consists of four main layers, which show a definite continuity throughout the hand.

Contracture of the superficial system produces interdigital contracture, and flexion of the proximal interphalangeal joints. The main result of contracture of the longitudinal layer has been found to be flexion of the metacarpophalangeal joints. The transverse

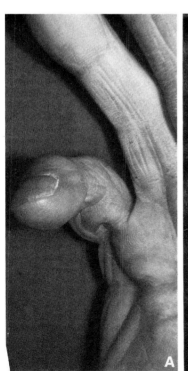
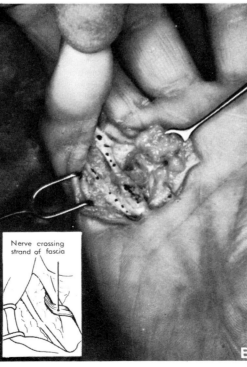

Figure 28.8
A, B, Dupuytren's contracture affecting the little finger.

fibres are seldom if ever involved. The anterior interosseous layer, continuous in the fingers with Cleland's ligaments, may be involved, causing contracture of the proximal interphalangeal joint.

There are several mechanisms of displacement of the digital nerves, and it has been found possible in a significant number of cases to predict when this displacement will occur, and thus reduce the risk of damage to the nerves during dissections to release the contractures.

ACKNOWLEDGEMENTS

My thanks are due to Professor Landsmeer for the opportunity to work in Leiden, and for permission to reproduce Figures 28.1 to 28.5, which were made by M. Bles. Figures 28.7 and 28.8 were photographed by R. F. Ruddick of The London Hospital.

I am also grateful to Dr K. M. Backhouse for the use of his material.

REFERENCES

ALLEN, H. S. (1954). Personal communication.

BROCK, R. C. (1952). *The Life and Work of Astley Cooper*, p. 150. Edinburgh: Livingstone.

CLELAND, J. (1878). Journal of Anatomy and Physiology, **12**, 526.

COOPER, A. P. (1822). *A Treatise on Dislocation and Fractures of the Joints*, 1st edn., p. 524.

DUPUYTREN, G. (1832). *Leçons Orales de Clinique Chirurgicales* faites à l'Hotel Dieu, vol. 1, p. 1. Paris: Ballière.

GOSSET, J. (1966). *Maladie de Dupuytren, Groupe d'Etude de la Main*, p. 15. Paris: L'Expansion Scientifique Française.

GRAPOW, M. (1887). *Archiv für Anatomie und Physiologie, Leipsig*, **2–3**, 143.

HUESTON, J. T. (1963). *Dupuytren's Contracture*. Edinburgh: Livingstone.

HUESTON, J. T. (1965). *Annals of the Royal College of Surgeons of England*, **36**, 134.

ISELIN, M. (1955). Chirurgie de la Main, Livre de Chirurgien. Paris: Masson et Cie.

LANDSMEER, J. M. F. (1956). *Compte rendu de l' Association des anatomistes*, **43**, 443.

LEGUEU, F. & JUVARA, E. (1892). *Bulletin de la Société anatomique de Paris*, 67th year, p. 383.

MASLIEURÀT-LAGÉMARD, G. E. (1839). *Gazette médicale de Paris*, **7/18**, 273.

NEZELOF, C. & TUBIANA, R. (1958). *Semaine des hôpitaux de Paris*, 34th year, **18/4**, 9.

PLÀTER, F. (1641). *Observationum*, Vol. 1, p. 150. Basel: König.

SKOOG, T. (1967). Scandinavian Journal of Plastic and Reconstructive Surgery, **1**, 51.

THOMINE, J. M. (1965). *Annales de chirurgie plastique*, **10/3**, 194.

29. POINTS OF AGREEMENT AND MODERN TRENDS IN THE TREATMENT OF DUPUYTREN'S CONTRACTURE

Raoul Tubiana

Having collected this comprehensive set of articles on the treatment of Dupuytren's contracture, we must now attempt to draw some conclusions.

In our own article on the 'principles of surgical treatment in Dupuytren's contracture', we discussed the most controversial views and gave the reasons for *our* choice. But, even at the risk of repeating ourselves, we would like to end this monograph by summarizing those views which appear to be shared by the majority of authors:

1. Treatment in Dupuytren's contracture has two basic aims; restoration of function and prevention of recurrence. When these aims are incompatible, especially in advanced cases, restoring function will have immediate priority. However important it may be, prophylactic treatment to prevent recurrence is still erratic and must not jeopardize the functional result.

2. The treatment is essentially surgical. Most of the present surgical procedures in spite of their intentions are little more than symptomatic corrections of deformities, and cannot hope to cure a systemic disease the nature of which is still poorly understood. Surgery has its limitations, and therefore one should not be mislead by overly optimistic statistics.

However, surgery can correct the majority of retraction deformities and, if well planned, can prevent most of the complications of the disease. If required it can even be repeated. While it is not exactly a panacaea, surgery remains the best form of treatment, but it must not prevent the development of new therapeutic approaches.

3. Under certain conditions, which require further elucidation, a simple fasciotomy may produce regression of the fibrous lesions, possibly due to suppression of longitudinal tension. A partical fasciectomy may have the same effect. In some cases however, surgical trauma appears to accelerate the evolution of the disease.

4. For a long time, the accent has been mainly on the treatment of palmar aponeurotic lesions. This concept should now be revised:

(a) without repeating the controversy concerning the initial localization of the lesions, it must now be accepted that these lesions spread beyond the aponeurotic formations, that the various aponeurotic structures are affected to different degrees, and that the dermis and subcutaneous tissue are often invaded. In addition, when the lesions are advanced there is secondary retraction of the capsule and ligaments of the digital joints and of the fibrous flexor tendon sheaths.

(b) Just as the lesions are not restricted to the aponeurosis nor are they restricted to the palm. In fact fibrosis lesions in the fingers resulting in retractions at the level of the interphalangeal joints carry a worse prognosis than palmar lesions which result in M.P. retractions which can be more easily corrected. As recurrences are much more frequent in the fingers and distal part of the palm, it is logical that surgical excision should be extended far into the affected fingers and their base, rather than into the rest of the palm. Transverse palmar incisions, which give good exposure of the palm but fail to display the danger zones where most of the lesions lie, must therefore be discarded in the majority of cases. Longitudinal digitopalmar incisions appear to be more suitable. In other words, surgical interest is no longer only fixed on palmar lesions, but seems to be more and more directed towards extra-aponeurotic lesions and towards the fingers.

5. Also the accent now tends to be on prevention, not only of recurrences, but above all of surgical complications. These represent a more immediate danger and may well delay functional recovery or sometimes leave the hand worse than before. There is, no doubt, a correlation between surgical complications and the severity of retractions, but more frequently such complications arise from faulty surgical indications such as overly extensive surgery in advanced cases.

It is well known that complications are more common after extended fasciectomies than after limited operations, but not in the proportion that one would expect. The commonest complications, haematomas, skin necrosis and joint stiffness are usually due to extensive undermining of the skin, incomplete haemostasis, unsuitable incisions and flaps, or to inadequate postoperative care. Most of these can be avoided. The experience of the surgeon and his attention to detail play an important part in preventing these complications.

6. The skin must be treated with the same thorough care as the aponeurosis. Poorly planned incisions and faulty closure are responsible for the majority of complications. It is probably better not to suture the teguments and allow secondary healing than to close the wound under tension or entrap a haematoma.

7. It is now generally accepted: (a) that a recurrence

may originate in the dermis; (b) that by excising the affected teguments and performing a skin graft, it may be possible to delay or even to prevent recurrences.

8. Recurrences seem to depend on several factors: (a) 'Dupuytren's contracture diathesis' which has been well described by J. Hueston.
(b) On the extent of fasciectomy, although this appears to be related more to the 'extension' of lesions rather than to the incidence of 'true recurrences' (recurrence in previously operated areas). Skin grafting has a preventive action which appears to block the development of recurrences. The reason for this has yet to be demonstrated: is it because some of the components of the transplanted skin, e.g. its nerve endings, have undergone degeneration, or because the graft is taken from a part of the body where Dupuytren's contracture never occurs and is of a 'different quality'?

9. All the facts tend to suggest that no single form of Dupuytren's contracture exists responding to one form of treatment. Treatment must be selective at all stages and, in every case, one must take into account the age of the patient, the possible aetiological factors, the site and extent of fascial involvement, and the state of the skin and joints.

10. Finally, one should not use the 'mysterious' nature of this disease as an excuse for avoiding further investigation, or as a convenient explanation for poor therapeutic results. The latter are usually due to faulty indications or poor technique.

AUTHOR INDEX

Abbe, R., 35
Adams, W., 49
Aron, E., 149
Barron, J., 99
Barclay, T., 123
Bassot, J., 31, 32
Beare, R., 79
Benassayag, R., 149–151
Berger, P., 74, 120
Boyes, J., 30, 69
Bruner, J. M., 93–94
Bunnell, S., 43, 64
Burch, P. R., 40
Carter, 37
Clarkson, P., 35, 43, 63–66, 119
Cline, H., 63
Conway, H., 63
Cooper, A., 63
Curtis, R. M., 135–137
Dabrowski, T., 29, 33, 35
Davis, J. E., 34
Dupuytren, G., 43, 63, 64
Early, P. F., 37, 38, 40, 43, 64
Ehlers, M., 70
Fisk, G., 43–44
Gonzalez, R., 30, 32, 75, 123–127, 143
Gordon, S., 64, 75, 120, 123
Gosset, J., 11–22, 30, 32, 72, 102
Goyrand, G., 11, 63, 111

Graubard, D. J., 64
Hakstian, R. W., 30, 59, 79–83
Hamlin, E., 123
Hassler, G., 30, 54
Herzog, E. G., 64
Howard, L., 69, 123
Hueston, J. T., 25, 27, 29–36, 38, 40, 43, 45, 49, 55, 58, 61–62, 63, 64, 65, 72, 73, 75, 76, 82, 85, 101, 111, 115, 119–122, 123, 126, 135, 141–147, 163
Iselin, M., 65, 67–70
Iselin, S., 139
James, J. I. P., 29, 37–42, 64
Kanabel, A. B., 130
Kaplin, E., 109
Kauffman, M. S., 32
Kvicala, V., 35
Lagier, 26
Landsmeer, J. M. F., 162
Larsen, R. D., 53, 112
Le Chuiton, M., 49
Lexer, E., 71, 120
Ling, R. S. M., 29, 37, 38, 39, 40, 41
Littler, J. W., 97–100
Luck, J. V., 31, 35, 71
Lund, M., 40, 64
MacCallum, P., 64, 111
McCash, C. R., 75, 91, 129–133
McIndoe, A. H., 49, 59, 79, 97, 112, 115
Mir-y-Mir, L., 75, 120
Michon, J., 45–47, 101–107

Millesi, H., 30, 31, 33, 45, 49–60, 72, 73, 81
Moorhead, J. J., 43, 49
Morley, G., 44
Moser, E., 49
Nauck, E., 50
Nezelof, C., 25–27, 35, 53, 72
Peacock, E., 32
Piulach, S., 75, 120
Plater, F., 63
Plewes, L., 43
Posch, J. L., 53, 112
Pulvertaft, G., 63, 64
Rang, M., 43
Rank, B. K., 64
Reid, D. C., 63, 64
Shaw, M. H., 73, 95–96, 123
Skoog, T., 26, 27, 32, 33, 40, 41, 51, 53, 65, 72, 109–117, 123
Stack, H. G., 32, 58, 153–162
Stin, A., 105
Straub, L. R., 32
Takagishi, N., 111
Thieme, W. T., 29, 39, 40, 41
Thomine, J. M., 1–9, 32, 69, 85–92
Tubiana, R., 25, 30, 35, 45–47, 53, 71–77, 85–92, 102, 163–164
Verso, M., 64
Williams, J., 149
Winklemann, R., 35
Wolfe, S. J., 119, 120
Zachariae, L., 70

SUBJECT INDEX

Abductor digiti minimi band, 61, 89, 99, 102
Activity rate, 54, 55
Aetiology, 27–64
  epilepsy, 39, 40, 43
  genetic, 37–42
  immobilization, 44
  neural factors, 35, 64
  role of alcohol, 35, 43, 61
  role of dermis, 36
  role of tension, 31–32
  role of vasomotor, 35
  trauma, 43–44
  vascularity, 35
Age incidence, 37, 43, 63, 64
  onset, 37, 50, 61, 79
Alcoholism, 35, 43, 61, 64
Amputation, 104, 137
  designation in staging, 46
Anaesthesia, 85, 131
  hypotensive, 73, 91
Animal experiments, 111

Aponeurosis, palmar
  anatomy, 1–9, 11–23, 58, 81, 88, 99, 109, 153–162
  changes with age, 50–84
    superficial transverse metacarpal ligament deep transverse fibres, 26, 33, 35, 51, 72, 109, 156
  development, 1, 154
  earliest macroscopic changes, 50, 72
  excision of, 87
  in relation to displacement of digital nerves, 68, 72, 99
  relationship to nodule, 26, 33, 72
  retrovascular band, 72
  segmentalization for staging, 45
Auto immunity hypothesis, 81

Bandages, 69
Blood group, 64
Brachial plexus block, 85, 97
Brewery workers, 43, 64

Callosity, 26, 146
Capsular contractures, 76, 137

Capsulotomy, 76, 102
  technique, 135–137
Classification,
  according to stage, 45
  according to histology, 53
Collagen
  role in contracture, 32, 49, 50–53, 81, 82
Compensation
  industrial and relationship, 43
Complications of surgery, 57, 58, 69–70, 73, 75, 80, 103
  and evaluation of results, 55
Course, 64
  clinical and morphological, 49–60, 79
  phasic nature, 54, 58

Deformity, evaluation of, 45–47
Dermal involvement, 26, 72
Dermis, role in aetiology, 32, 35, 36, 72
Diathesis, 30, 35, 54, 61, 73, 85, 120, 145
Digital nerve,
  displacement, 67, 68, 72, 99, 112
  injury, 67, 68, 72, 74
Distribution of disease, 123

Dressings, 69, 73, 74, 91, 99, 131

Ectopic deposits
  histology, 26, 33
  incidence, 30, 145
  management, 146
  prognostic significance, 61, 73
  sites,
    forearm, 30
    general, 61
    gingival, 30
    knuckle pads, 25, 30, 43, 65, 146
    penile, 43, 54, 146
    plantar, 30, 43
    tendo achilles, 30, 145
Epileptics
  incidence, 29, 39, 40, 43, 44
  penile lesions, 65
  prognosis, 61
Extension of disease process, 32, 55, 61, 65
  definition, 46, 55, 72

Family history, 37, 43, 61
Fasciectomy
  complications
    finger necrosis, 104
    haematoma, 73, 99, 103
    intrinsic plus, 106
    oedema, 73, 104
    Sudek's atrophy, 105
  limited, 62, 76, 123
    results, 49, 55
  open palm technique, 131
  radical, 62, 71
    results, 49, 55, 72, 73, 79–83
    technique, 86–92, 95, 97
  with wolfe graft, 62, 76, 99, 119, 120
Fasciotomy
  enzymic, 31, 41–143
  open, 61, 71, 75, 85
  subcutaneous, 30, 32, 49
  with wolfe graft, 30, 123–127
Fat replacement, 25, 26, 27, 32, 33, 65
Foreign body significance, 32
Formulae for staging, 45–47

Genetic factors, 29, 37–42, 43, 81
Grafts
  distant flap, 91, 99, 101, 119, 137
  local flap, 69, 91, 97, 101
  wolfe graft, 30, 32, 35, 62, 74, 99, 101,
    115, 119, 123

Haematoma, 57, 91, 99, 103
Haemorrhage,
  interstitial, 53
  microscopic, 27
Handedness and incidence, 43, 44
Heredity, 29, 43, 44, 37–42, 61, 63
Histology, 25–27, 49–53, 81
  collagen fibres, 25, 32
  ectopic lesions, 145
  interphalangeal bands, 25
  knuckle pads, 25, 33
  lamellar form, 25, 50, 81
  nodular form, 25, 50, 81
  palmar nodules, 25, 33
  skin involvement, 26, 72

Hueston's extrinsic theory, 27, 33
Hyperplastic structure, 25, 32, 50–53
Hypertrophy of bands, 35, 61, 65

Incidence
  age, 29, 37, 50
  alcoholics, 35, 43
  barbiturates, 29, 41
  epileptics, 29, 40, 43
  handedness, 43, 44
  invalids, 35
  manual and non manual workers, 43–44
  racial, 29, 38
  sex, 38
  tuberculosis, 43
Incisions, 57, 69, 74, 85, 86, 87, 93, 95, 97,
    101, 115, 131, 135
Injury, relation to, 32, 35, 43–44, 53
Interphalangeal band, 25, 61
Interphalangeal joints
  distal
    flexion deformity, 61, 76
    hyperextension deformity, 61, 65, 89
    relation to staging deformity, 45, 56
  proximal
    capsular contractures, 76, 137
    collateral ligament changes, 76, 102
    correction of deformity, 90, 91, 102
    in staging deformity, 45, 56
    uncontrollable deformity, 76, 77, 124,
      135
Iron pigment, 27, 53

Joints
  interphalangeal, *see* Interphalangeal
    joints
  metacarpophalangeal
    correction, 61
    in staging deformity, 45, 46

Knuckle pads
  excision, 146
  histology, 25, 33, 145
  incidence, 30, 65, 145
  prognostic significance, 30, 61, 65, 145
  recurrence, 147

Macroscopic appearance, 33, 50, 71
Metaplasia, 33
Methylhydrazine in treatment of Peyronie's
  disease, 149–151
Micro haemorrhages, 27, 53
Micro ruptures, fascial, 27, 53, 111
Microscopic appearances, *see* Histology
Mitotic figures, 145

Natatory ligament, 5, 72, 95, 112
Natural history, 29, 30, 43, 49–60, 61, 64,
  68
Neuralgia, post-operative, 105
Night splints, 133
Nodules
  appearance, 33, 68
  histology, 25, 26, 27, 50–53
  role of, 32, 72
  site of origin, 33, 34, 50, 64, 65, 72

Occupation, relation to, 43–44

Oedema, post-operative, 57, 68, 73
Onset, 30, 49–60, 71

Pacinian corpuscles, 26, 36
Painful lesions, 65
Palmar aponeurosis, *see* Aponeurosis,
  palmar
Pathogenesis, 34–36, 49–60, 81, 109, 111
Penile lesions, 43, 61, 65
Periarthritis humeri, 43
Perivascular changes, 52
Peyronie's disease, 65, 146, 147, 149
  treatment, 146, 149
Plantar lesions, 65, 145
  excision of, 146
  histology of, 33, 145
  incidence of, 30, 145
  prognostic significance, 30, 61, 145
  recurrence, of, 147
Plasma proteins, 70
Post-operative framboesial palmar fibrosis,
  64
Post-operative management
  complications, 57, 69, 80
  recurrence, 30, 31, 49, 55, 62
  stiffness, 69
  swelling, 57, 69
  tenderness, 80
Progression, 30, 45, 49–60, 64
Prognosis
  pre-operative assessment of, 45, 55, 61
  general and local factors in, 61
Psychiatric aspects, 70

Racial factors, 29, 30, 38, 63, 64
Recurrence
  definition, 46, 55, 72, 139
  'false recurrence', 67, 139
  incidence, 31, 39
  prevention by wolfe graft, 32, 35, 62, 75,
    119
  significance of, 36, 55, 73, 106
  time of, 30, 58, 73
Results, general, 55, 57, 105
  of fasciectomy, 31, 49, 55
  of limited fasciectomy, 31, 49, 55, 62,
    106, 123
  of radical fasciectomy, 31, 49, 56, 62, 79,
    105
  of enzymic fasciotomy, 31
Retinacular ligament, 89, 102, 135
Retrovascular band, 72, 89

Secondary surgery, 61, 107
Sensory disturbances, 65
Sex incidence, 38, 39, 43, 61, 63, 79
Skin covering, 74, 91
Skin involvement
  biopsies, 26
  skin pits, 34
Staging deformity, 45–47, 54
  histologically, 51–53
Subcutaneous palmar space, 35, 36
Sudek's atrophy, relation to, 43, 69, 104

Tendon sheath involvement, 63, 75, 90,
  102, 135
Tennis elbow, relation to, 43

Tension, role of, 32, 33, 65
Thumb involvement, 61, 63
  in staging deformity, 45
  treatment, 86, 89
Tourniquet, use of, 85, 93, 97, 131
Trauma, relation to, 43–44, 53, 63, 64, 65, 81, 112
Tuberculosis, incidence in pulmonary, 43

Twins, incidence in, 43, 145
Theory
  intrinsic, 33, 49–60, 111, 146
  extrinsic, 33, 146

Ulnar nerve damage, 64

Vascularaity of palmar tissues, 25, 34, 35

Vasomotor changes, 35, 36

Web contractures, and digital nerve, 68
Wolfe grafts, 30, 32, 61
Women, incidence in, 38, 39, 43, 79

Z-plastic rearrangement of skin, 74, 86, 89, 90, 91, 93, 96, 97, 112, 115, 135

PRINTED IN GREAT BRITAIN
by T. & A. Constable Ltd, Edinburgh